Table of Contents

DIABETES RENAL DIET COOKBOOK

For Seniors

The Complete Seniors' Low Carb Guide to Managing Kidney Disease and Diabetes with 100+ Nourishing Recipes

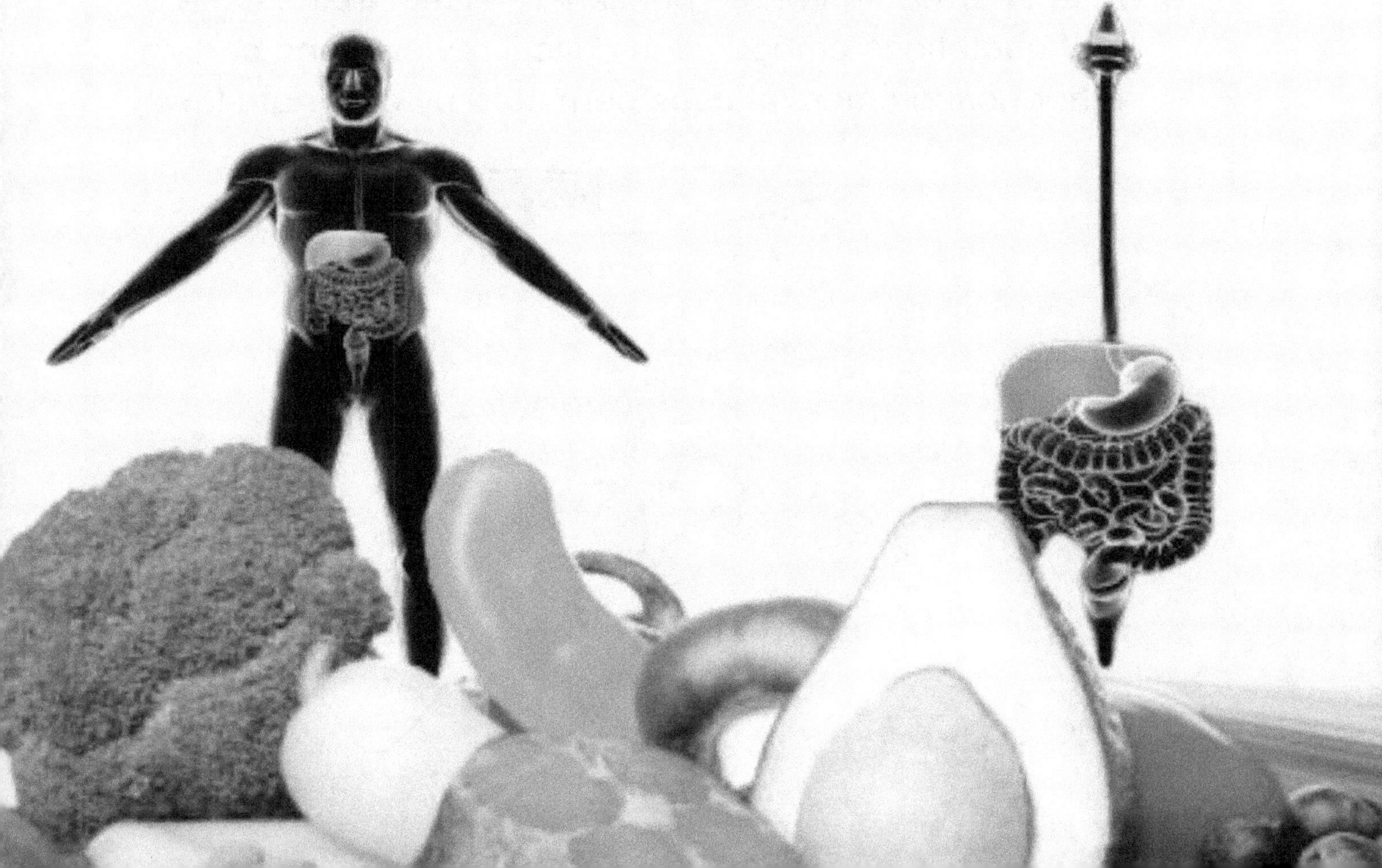

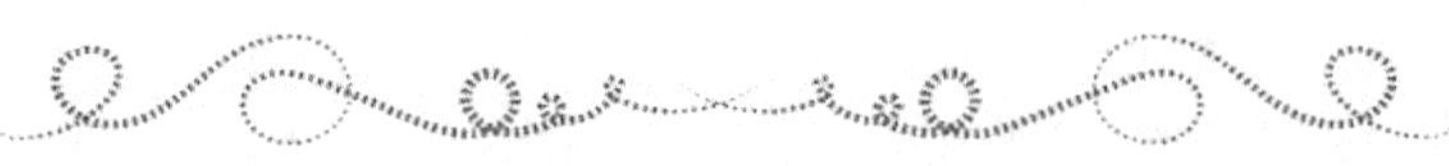

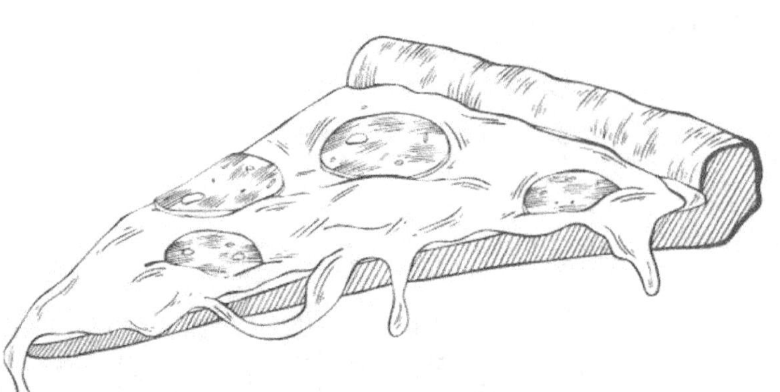

Copyright © 2024 VIVIAN GREENE

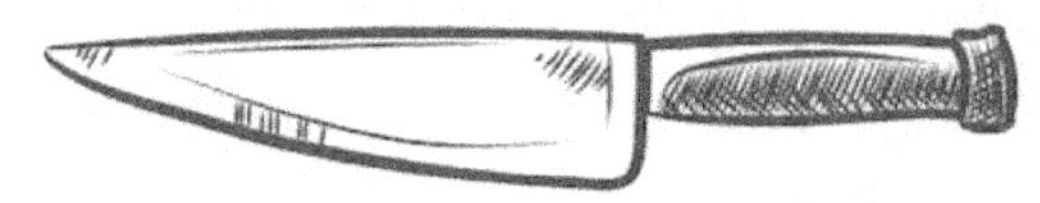

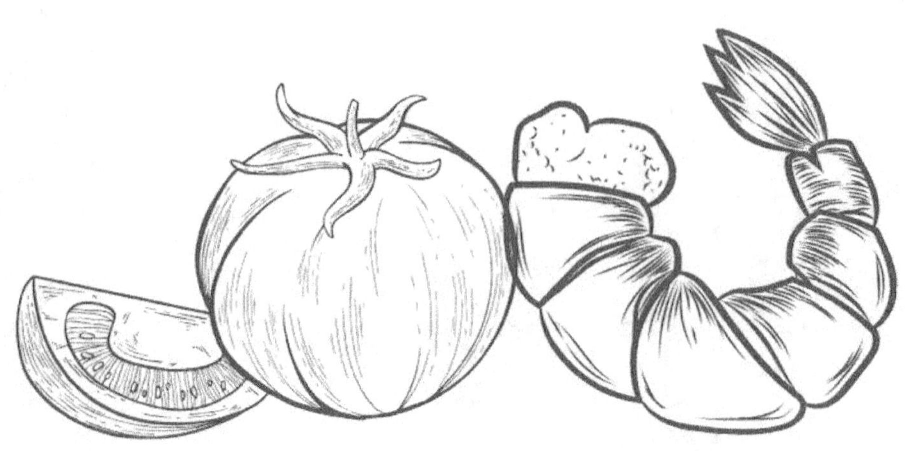

Introduction

As a seasoned writer and health advocate, I've had the honor of seeing numerous people successfully negotiate the complex web of health issues, especially when it comes to the confluence of diabetes and renal disease, especially in our dear elderly. One theme keeps coming up in the patchwork of tales I've read: the urgent need for comprehension and practical advice.

Imagine an elderly room full of people who are all juggling the weight of renal disease and diabetes. Their tales read like worn-out book pages, with every chapter replete with victories, disappointments, and an unwavering will to live life to the fullest. This compelling story makes the need for a customized approach to health abundantly evident.

It is undoubtedly difficult to manage renal disease and diabetes together. A careful balance is needed to perform the complex dance of controlling blood sugar levels, following dietary limitations, and preserving general well-being. But in my interactions with these strong people, I've seen an incredible shift—a resolute determination to take control of their health, bolstered by knowledge and the desire to fully enjoy life.

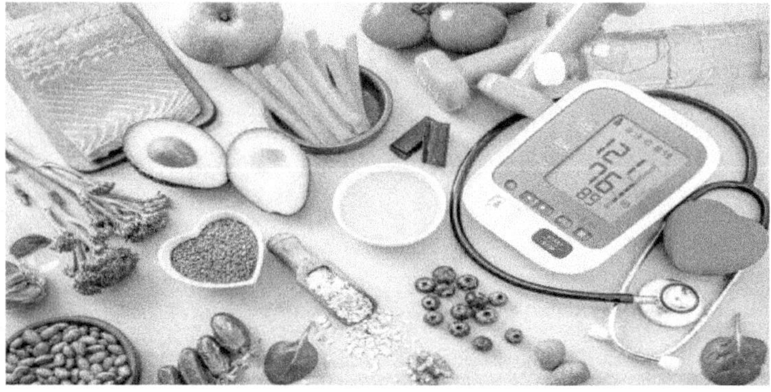

The combined knowledge gained from these experiences is embodied in this book, "Diabetes Renal Diet Cookbook for Seniors: The Complete Seniors' Low Carb Guide to Managing Kidney Disease and Diabetes with 100+ Nourishing Recipes." For those navigating the complex maze of diabetes and renal illness, it is a lighthouse that offers not only a route map but also a traveling companion.

We will explore the nuances of various medical illnesses on these pages, using firsthand accounts and true tales to highlight the difficulties older people have. Together, we will investigate the life-changing potential of a low-carb, renal-friendly diet—a gastronomic adventure that satisfies the palate while nourishing the body.

In addition to spreading knowledge, as a specialist in health and wellbeing, my mission is to craft a story that will appeal to every reader. We're going to take a trip that explores the core of human experience, going beyond clinical language. I want to inspire every elder, caregiver, and health enthusiast to embrace a life of energy and pleasure despite the challenges posed by diabetes and renal disease through the tales I tell and the useful advice I provide.

Together, let's go off on this journey, turning the pages of information with excitement rather than fear, as a brighter, healthier future lies ahead.

The relationship between diabetes and renal disease is a complicated nexus that requires our understanding and attention in the complex web of senior health. As we explore the subtleties of these diseases, it becomes clear that negotiating this cohabitation with our beloved elders takes customized knowledge that goes beyond traditional health information.

Let's start by examining the complexities of diabetes, a disease that is becoming much more frequent among the elderly population. Seniors with diabetes, which is defined by high blood sugar, encounter several challenges. As people age, their body's capacity to either create or use insulin decreases, making it more difficult for seniors to maintain their blood sugar levels. Uncontrolled diabetes may cause a host of other health problems that can impair essential organs and lower one's quality of life in general.

The stakes are much higher when renal illness is added to this story. The kidneys are essential to preserving the body's delicate equilibrium because they filter waste and extra fluid from circulation. However, diabetes presents a serious risk to these essential organs, especially if left unchecked. The illness known as diabetic nephropathy, which is characterized by a progressive decline in kidney function, is caused by a compromise of the complex system of blood vessels inside the kidneys.

This dual diagnosis often signals a time of uncertainty and adjustment for elders. Diabetic problems add to the already heavy weight that aging has placed on the kidneys. Seniors with diabetes have a markedly increased risk of renal damage, which makes proactive holistic health care necessary.

The education component of this proactive strategy is crucial. Seniors who are caring for others need to be aware of the mutually beneficial association between diabetes and renal illness. It's critical to recognize the warning signs and symptoms of both disorders. Uncontrolled diabetes may be the cause of symptoms including increased thirst, frequent urination, and unexplained weight loss. Conversely, altered urine color, chronic tiredness, and ankle edema may indicate impaired kidney function.

For seniors with diabetes and renal illnesses, routine monitoring becomes essential. Vital signs such as blood pressure, renal function tests, and blood sugar levels are monitored closely in this watchful manner. Equipped with this data, medical practitioners may customize therapies that cater to the distinct requirements of every senior, therefore slowing down the advancement of these ailments.

Beyond the therapeutic setting, lifestyle changes are essential for enabling elders to take charge of their health. A low-carb, well-balanced diet is the key to treating renal disease and diabetes. Elderly people are urged to go on a gastronomic adventure that not only meets their dietary requirements but also takes into account the limitations placed on them by these circumstances.

We will examine the practical issues of putting such dietary modifications into practice in the next chapters of this book. Seniors will learn via a carefully chosen selection of more than 100 nutritional dishes that a low-carb, renal-friendly diet can be tasty and varied in addition to being health-conscious.

As we go out on this path of comprehension, let us acknowledge that empowerment is contingent upon knowledge. Understanding the complex relationship between diabetes and kidney disease in the elderly helps us make educated choices, take proactive measures to maintain our health, and eventually help our loved ones live longer, healthier lives.

Importance of a Renal Diet for Seniors with Diabetes

The combination of diabetes and renal illness creates a specific difficulty in the complex web of health, particularly for our beloved elderly. It is an honor for me to raise awareness of the critical role that a renal diet plays in the lives of seniors who are coping with both illnesses as an advocate for health and well-being.

We must first disentangle the symbiotic link between diabetes and kidney health in order to fully appreciate the relevance of a renal diet. Over time, diabetes, a disease marked by high blood sugar, may have a significant effect on the kidneys. The kidneys, which are in charge of eliminating waste and extra fluid from the blood, are most affected by this ongoing blood sugar rise. Diabetic nephropathy is a disorder caused by damage to the delicate filtering units inside the kidneys called nephrons.

Here comes the renal diet, a carefully planned dietary plan designed to reduce the burden on the kidneys and slow the advancement of kidney disease. Adopting a renal diet becomes an essential part of holistic health care for seniors who are already managing diabetes.

Control of certain nutrients, particularly salt and protein, is one of the main tenets of a renal diet for elderly people with diabetes. Oversoiling with salt may lead to fluid retention, which puts more strain on already-weakened kidneys. Seniors may lessen the burden on their kidneys and better control their blood pressure by consuming less salt. In addition, moderate protein consumption is essential as too much protein might worsen renal impairment. The renal diet creates a careful balance between giving seniors enough protein to feed them and keeping their kidneys from suffering needlessly.

The regulation of potassium and phosphorus in a renal diet is equally important. Mineral imbalances may have a disastrous effect on the body's delicate balance, especially in those with impaired renal function. The strategic approach of the renal diet provides comfort to older adults with diabetes by pointing them in the direction of dietary choices that facilitate internal system harmony rather than conflict.

Apart from the dietary complexities, another area in which a renal diet is beneficial is blood sugar regulation, which is crucial for diabetics. Seniors may efficiently control their diabetes while protecting the health of their kidneys by choosing complex carbs over simple ones. The mutually beneficial association between diabetes and kidney disease highlights the comprehensive approach of the renal diet, which attends to not a single element but rather the intricate network of health issues.

A renal diet has far-reaching effects that go far beyond just what happens at mealtimes. It turns into a way of life, an intentional decision to take care of the body and maintain the delicate equilibrium needed for optimum health. Seniors who go on this gastronomic adventure feel empowered by the knowledge that they can actively maintain their kidney function, which promotes well-being and a feeling of control.

it is impossible to exaggerate the significance of a renal diet for elderly people with diabetes. It serves as a compass to help people navigate the maze of health issues and provides them with both nourishment and a path back to vigor. Seniors may take a step towards improved well-being by adopting the principles of a renal diet. This will help them to enjoy life to the fullest even with the complications of diabetes and kidney disease. It's a harmonic tango between nutrition and health.

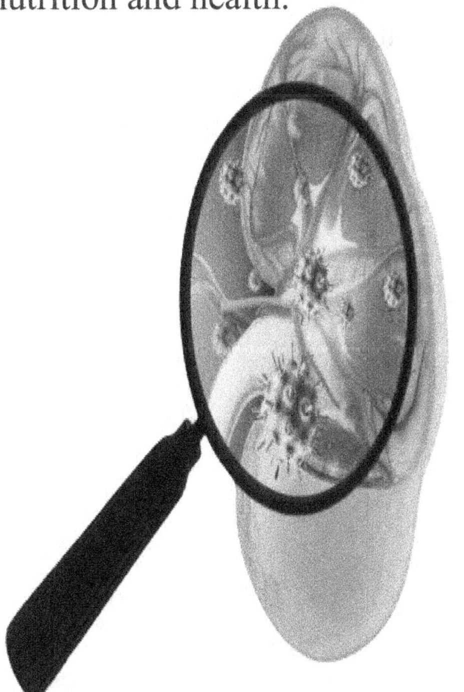

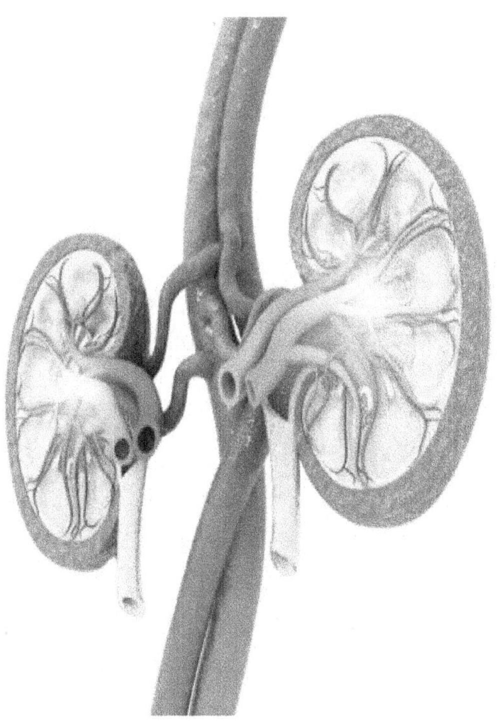

Chapter 1

BASICS OF DIABETES AND KIDNEY DISEASE

Overview of Diabetes in Seniors

The complicated dance with health evolves along with our journey through life's tapestry, and for many seniors, diabetes becomes an important companion in this complex waltz. Diabetes is a chronic illness that is defined by increased blood sugar levels. Its effects on the well-being of the senior population require comprehensive knowledge of this disease.

First and foremost, it's critical to understand that diabetes often presents differently in older adults than in younger ones. Aging may cause physiological changes that affect the body's glucose regulation. Type 2 diabetes is characterized by increased insulin resistance and decreased pancreatic insulin production. Seniors are more susceptible to issues associated with diabetes due to these variables.

The most common kind of diabetes in seniors is type 2, which is often associated with lifestyle choices including food and exercise. Diabetes may become more prevalent as a result of lifelong food and activity patterns that combine with genetic predispositions. Moreover, co-occurring medical disorders are often seen in the elderly population and might worsen the complications associated with diabetes, further complicating its care.

Diabetes complications are a serious risk to the health of elderly people. The increased risk of cardiovascular problems, such as heart disease and stroke, highlights the systemic effects of uncontrolled blood sugar levels. Seniors with diabetes may also develop neuropathy, retinopathy, and nephropathy, which emphasizes the need for comprehensive treatment that goes beyond glucose control.

Seniors with diabetes often have modest symptom presentations, so routine testing and education are crucial. Increased thirst, frequent urination, unexplained weight loss, and exhaustion are typical symptoms. However, other age-related illnesses may hide these signals, delaying diagnosis and perhaps causing consequences.

An all-encompassing strategy is necessary for the treatment of diabetes in the elderly. The cornerstones of optimal diabetic treatment include regular physical activity, dietary adjustments, and medication control. For long-term management to be effective, treatment programs must be customized to meet the specific requirements of elders, taking mobility and cognitive function into account.

Getting elders to practice self-care requires teamwork from caregivers and support systems in addition to medical experts. Education and empowerment are important because they help people understand the disease and provide them with the tools they need to handle it daily.

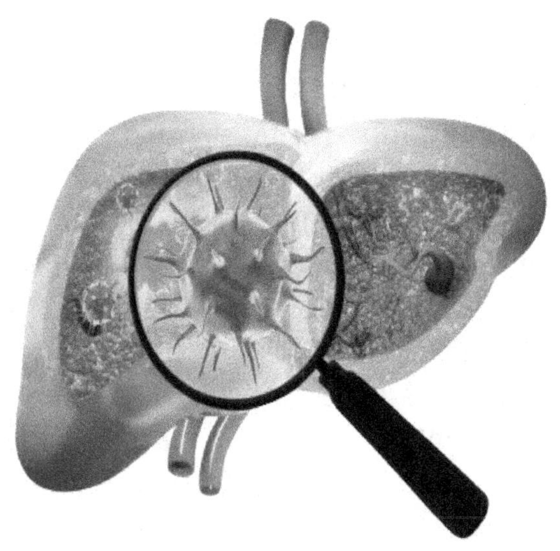

Few relationships in the complex web of human health are as significant and deep-rooted as the one between diabetes and renal disease. As a writer who is passionate about health and wellness, I have seen firsthand how this complex connection affects a great number of people's lives, especially when it comes to our beloved elders.

Let's set out to explore the nuances of kidney illness and how it coexists with diabetes, illuminating the physiological subtleties that highlight this sometimes difficult partnership.

Diabetes and Kidney Disease: A Quiet Collaboration

See your kidneys as the unsung warriors who quietly remove waste and extra fluid from your blood while maintaining a delicate balance that is essential for good health. Now superimpose the complex dance of diabetes, a disease marked by high blood sugar levels, over this picture. The relationship between renal illness and diabetes is formed within this delicate balance.

The circulatory system is the foundation of this partnership. Blood vessels all over the body might sustain damage from diabetes, particularly if it is not well controlled. The kidneys' microscopic blood vessels, which filter waste, are especially vulnerable to this attack. Kidney disease may begin when high blood sugar levels cause diabetic nephropathy, a disorder that progresses over time.

To manage the effects of diabetic kidney disease, it is essential to understand how the illness progresses. The story is told in phases, each distinguished by unique clinical traits:

Early Stage (Microalbuminuria): The kidneys begin to leak trace quantities of the protein albumin into the urine during this first stage. Even though there may not be any obvious symptoms, this is a warning indication of possible renal problems.

Intermediate Stage (Proteinuria): As the illness worsens, there is an increased leakage of albumin, which raises the amount of protein in the urine. The systemic character of the illness is shown by the fact that this stage often coexists with a rise in blood pressure.

Advanced Stage (End-Stage Renal Disease): End-stage renal disease (ESRD) is the last stage of diabetic kidney disease, which is characterized by a severe loss of kidney function. At this stage, the kidneys are no longer able to filter waste products efficiently, making dialysis or kidney transplantation necessary.

High blood sugar and high blood pressure

To understand the relationship between diabetes and kidney illness, we need to focus on the main causes, which are hyperglycemia (high blood sugar) and hypertension (high blood pressure).

Hyperglycemia: Extended periods of high blood sugar set off a series of reactions that aggravate kidney injury. The presence of too much glucose in the blood may aggravate kidney damage by causing oxidative stress, inflammation, and the activation of certain pathways.

Hypertension: Damage to blood vessels brought on by diabetes not only directly damages the kidneys but also increases the effects of hypertension. Renal illness advances more quickly when blood pressure is raised because it puts more strain on the kidneys' fragile filtering mechanism.

Prevention and Management

Although the confluence of diabetes and renal disease presents several obstacles, there is still hope. Proactive management, awareness, and education are essential for reducing the effects and guiding oneself in the direction of improved health.

Blood Sugar Control: One of the most important strategies to limit the course of diabetic kidney disease is to maintain ideal blood sugar levels through dietary changes, medication adherence, and routine monitoring.

Blood Pressure Management:

Maintaining renal function depends critically on controlling hypertension. Crucial elements of this method include medication adherence, lifestyle changes, and routine blood pressure readings.

Renal-Friendly Diet: It's crucial to follow a diet designed to promote kidney health. This entails eating a balanced, nutrient-rich diet, limiting the amount of protein you eat, and consuming less salt.

Diabetes and kidney illness are linked in a complex web of physiological interdependence. Using comprehension, consciousness, and anticipatory actions, people may maneuver this intricate terrain with fortitude and a strengthened feeling of authority. The route toward holistic health and well-being may be difficult, but armed with information as a guide, we can make sure that the complex dance between kidney disease and diabetes is performed with elegance and energy.

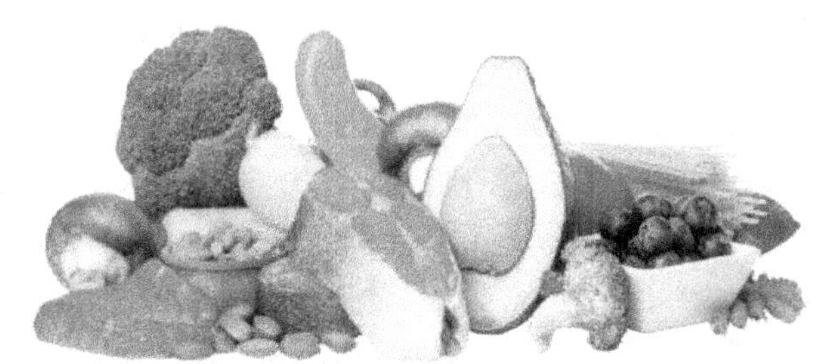

Complicated Medication Management: Seniors who struggle with diabetes and renal illness often get enmeshed in the complex world of prescription drugs. The difficulty is not only in knowing the function and dose of each treatment, but also in balancing the possibility of drug interactions between kidney health-protecting and diabetes-targeting medications. To guarantee a pharmaceutical regimen that is both safe and effective, careful cooperation between healthcare professionals becomes essential.

Dietary Decisions: Making wise dietary choices is essential to controlling diabetes and renal disease. There are many obstacles in the way of this journey, however. Sometimes the dietary guidelines for diabetes—which often call for close monitoring of carbohydrates—conflict with a renal diet, which emphasizes restricting certain nutrients to lessen the load on the kidneys. Seniors have to walk a tightrope, managing a variety of dietary limitations while making sure they are getting enough nourishment to suit their particular health requirements.

Blood Sugar Rollercoaster: Diabetes and kidney illness have a synergistic connection that makes for a precarious blood sugar rollercoaster. Blood sugar swings may make renal problems worse, resulting in a difficult cycle that needs close observation. In addition to controlling their food consumption, seniors may also need to manage their stress levels, physical exercise, and medication adherence to maintain blood sugar stability.

Fluid management: The body's fluid balance is often upset by kidney illness, which may result in consequences including edema and elevated blood pressure. Seniors who have renal disease or diabetes must manage their fluid intake carefully since these two illnesses need careful attention to hydration. Finding the ideal balance becomes essential, necessitating elders to watch how much liquids they drink while taking blood sugar and renal function into account.

Cognitive Health Issues: Diabetes and renal disease have complex interactions that affect cognitive health in addition to physical health. Seniors may have cognitive issues, such as memory loss and focus problems. Their quest for better health management may become even more complicated as a result of this cognitive fog, which may make it difficult for them to follow prescription regimens, check blood sugar levels, and make wise food decisions.

Limited Physical Activity: Diabetes and renal illness together often cause low energy and impaired physical capabilities. Seniors may find themselves in a predicament where the weariness and physical restrictions brought on by renal disease collide with the need of consistent physical exercise for managing diabetes. It becomes difficult to find a balance between being mobile and preventing overexertion.

It is certainly a difficult undertaking to navigate the complicated terrain of controlling renal disease and diabetes in seniors. However, the difficulties provide a chance for resiliency and change. Seniors who have a thorough understanding of the complexities of medication management, dietary subtleties, blood sugar control, fluid balance, cognitive health, and physical exercise are more equipped to make educated choices and feel more in charge of their health.

Let's keep in mind that every difficulty we face may lead to development, resilience, and the prospect of living a better, more fulfilling life as we explore the world of these prevalent problems. Seniors may take a journey that transcends the complexity of multiple conditions and embraces a future characterized by vitality, pleasure, and empowered well-being using education, support, and a holistic approach to health.

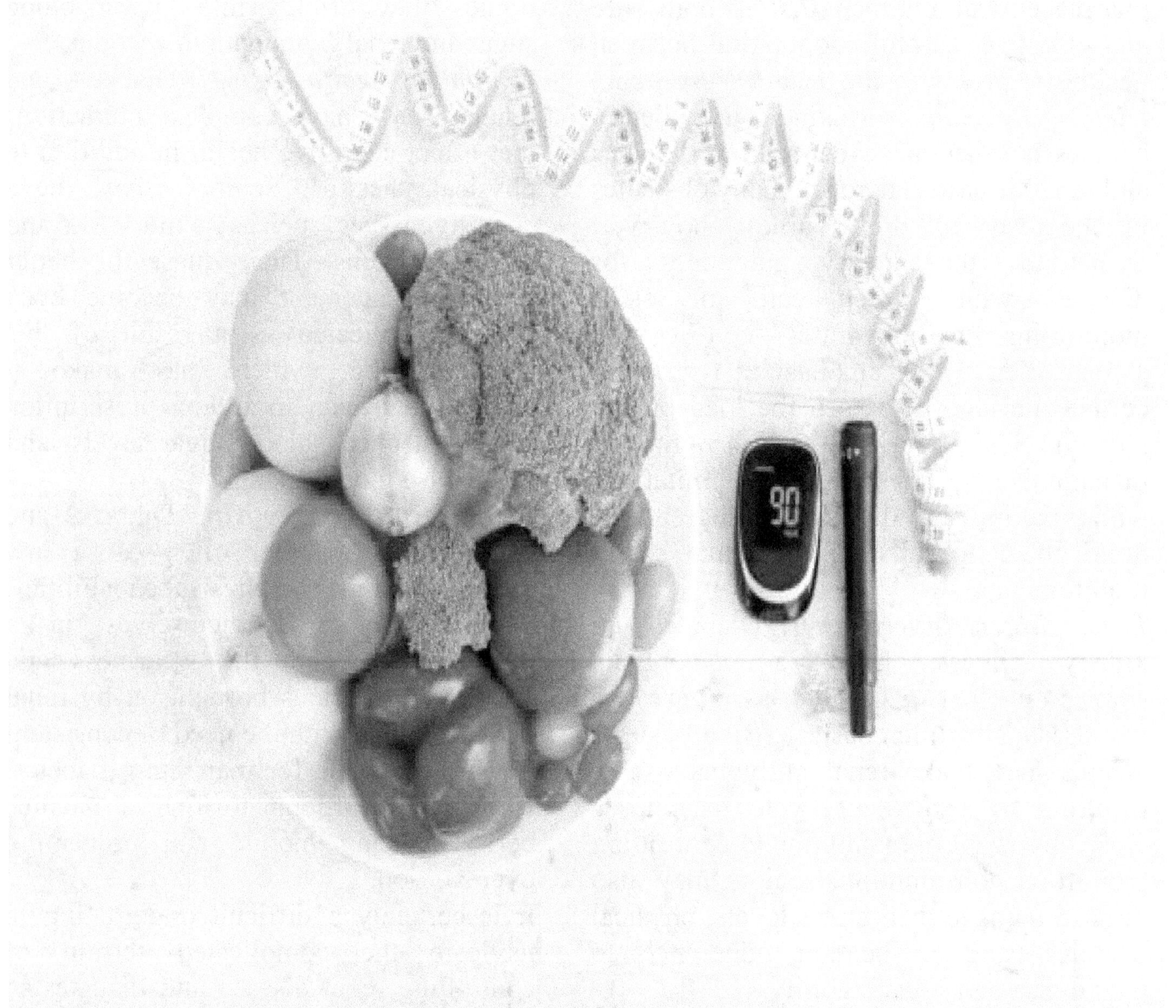

Chapter 2

SENIORS' LOW CARB GUIDE

Benefits of a Low Carb Diet for Seniors

Within the array of nutritional approaches, the notion of a low-carb diet has become a potent ally, especially for older adults juggling the twin burdens of diabetes and renal disease. The more we explore the complex landscape of health, the more clear it is that a low-carb diet has advantages well beyond helping with weight loss. Let's explore the nuances of why a low-carb diet is so beneficial to senior health.

1. Blood Sugar Control: A low-carb diet's significant effect on blood sugar levels is one of the main benefits for seniors who follow it. For those with diabetes, carbohydrates—especially refined sugars—can result in sharp rises in blood glucose that present serious challenges. Seniors may benefit from more stable blood sugar levels and improved glycemic control by consuming less carbohydrates. This promotes general well-being in addition to lowering the risk of complications from diabetes.

2. Weight Management: Seniors sometimes struggle to maintain a healthy weight due to the natural slowing down of their metabolism. In this way, a low-carb diet may make a difference. Reducing the amount of carbohydrates consumed encourages the body to utilize fat reserves for energy, which aids in weight reduction. Furthermore, seniors may feel fuller for longer periods because of the natural satiety that comes with a diet high in proteins and healthy fats, which may reduce needless snacking and support a long-term approach to weight control.

3. Better Cardiovascular Health: Seniors who may be more vulnerable to heart-related problems should place a high priority on their cardiovascular health. Numerous cardiovascular risk variables are favorably impacted by a low-carb diet. People may have decreased blood pressure, better HDL (good) cholesterol, and lowered triglyceride levels by consuming less refined carbs. By improving cardiovascular health overall, these advantages lower the chance of heart disease.

4. Improved Kidney Function: Diet and kidney health are closely related to seniors who are coping with diabetes and renal illness. Because a low-carb diet minimizes the effort that comes with digesting large quantities of carbs, it is naturally gentler on the kidneys. Seniors may be able to slow down the course of kidney disease and eventually improve renal function by lessening the stress on their kidneys.

5. Aging and Cognitive Health: Concerns about aging-related neurodegenerative illnesses and cognitive impairment are often voiced by seniors. There may be a connection between cognitive health and carbohydrate intake, according to recent studies. By supporting brain health, a low-carb diet may protect against age-related cognitive decline. It is thought that the ketones generated when lipids are broken down for energy have neuroprotective qualities, which may lower the risk of diseases like Alzheimer's.

6. Controlling Inflammation: Diabetes and renal disease are two conditions that are shared by several age-related illnesses, such as chronic inflammation. It has been shown that a low-carb diet contains anti-inflammatory properties, which may lower the body's inflammatory indicators. Seniors may benefit from problems made worse by chronic inflammation by reducing inflammatory processes, which will enhance their quality of life.

7. Stable Energy Levels: Elderly people often talk about how their energy levels fluctuate, which affects their daily activities and general vigor. A low-carb diet helps maintain energy levels throughout the day by giving fats and proteins a consistent source of energy. Seniors' capacity to participate in physical activities may be improved by this prolonged energy release, encouraging an active and satisfying lifestyle.

A low-carb diet has many advantages for seniors that go far beyond helping them lose weight. Adopting a low-carb strategy may be a game-changer for overall health, having positive effects on everything from inflammation management and cognitive function to blood sugar regulation and cardiovascular health. Let a low-carb diet's ease of use and effectiveness guide us through the complexities of aging, leading to a happy and satisfying trip.

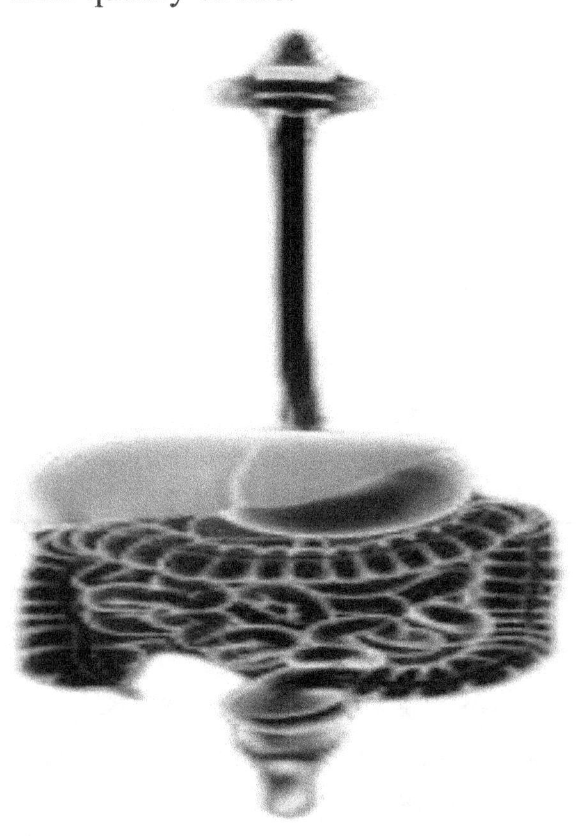

Two important pillars stand tall in the complex web of treating diabetes: measuring carbohydrates and closely monitoring blood sugar levels. These practices are more than just routines for those who are dealing with this illness; they are essential resources that enable them to take charge of their health and well-being. Together, we will explore the science behind blood sugar monitoring and carb counting, as well as their tremendous effects. Let's go on this trip to discover these practices' transformational potential.

Counting Carbs: Solving the Dietary Mysteries

A staple of the human diet, carbohydrates may be found in a variety of foods such as bread, rice, pasta, fruits, and vegetables. Since the body's capacity to control blood sugar is compromised in diabetics, it is essential to watch and control the amount of carbohydrates consumed.

Counting carbohydrates is an empowering method that empowers people to make educated decisions about their diet. By not looking at eating as a means of limitation, this method encourages flexibility and self-control. People who are aware of how much carbs are in different foods may adjust their meals to keep their blood sugar levels steady.

Picture an older citizen with diabetes equipped with the knowledge of carb counting and navigating the grocery store aisles. They make decisions that are in line with their health objectives with confidence rather than feeling overwhelmed. It's important to make decisions that support balance and well-being rather than completely cutting up carbs.

Furthermore, meal planning with a sophisticated approach is encouraged by carb counting. It promotes knowledge of how various carbs affect blood sugar levels, enabling the preparation of well-balanced meals. This information is more than just statistics; it offers a method for people to have a more positive connection with food and enjoy meals that satisfy their bodies and spirits.

The Harmony of Blood Sugar Tracking

Blood sugar levels are like the body's internal symphony; they need to be carefully adjusted to keep health at its best. This symphony may sometimes be dissonant for those with diabetes, necessitating close observation to guarantee harmony.

Frequent blood sugar monitoring gives you real-time data on how your body reacts to different stimulants like food, exercise, and medications. It's similar to fine-tuning an instrument. Preventing hypo- and hyperglycemia by maintaining blood sugar levels within a specific range is the main objective.

Blood sugar monitoring is now a smoother and more user-friendly experience, thanks to modern technologies. Real-time data from blood glucose meters and continuous glucose monitors (CGMs) enables people to make prompt lifestyle modifications. As watchful protectors, these gadgets notify users when their blood sugar levels stray from the target range.

Consider a senior who uses technology as an ally in their quest for health and skillfully incorporates blood sugar monitoring into their everyday routine. Empowerment and well-informed decision-making are more important than merely statistics on a screen. Regular monitoring helps people see trends, comprehend the peculiar reactions of their bodies, and work well with medical specialists to improve the way they manage their diabetes.

The Interdependence of Blood Sugar Monitoring and Carbohydrate Counting

Blood sugar monitoring and carb counting work together to create a symbiotic connection that enables people to control their diabetes. While blood sugar monitoring gives real-time data on the body's reaction to dietary choices, carb counting provides the road map for those decisions.

This synergy is not limited to the therapeutic setting; it is woven throughout everyday existence. It's the satisfaction that comes from enjoying a nutritious meal and seeing the glucose monitor's readings match your health objectives. It's the assurance that comes from being aware of how dietary habits affect blood sugar levels and having the ability to make decisions without fear.

Essentially, blood sugar monitoring and carb counting are roads to a life of empowerment and well-being rather than just habits. Let's welcome these tools with open arms as we negotiate the complex terrain of diabetes care, realizing their transforming power in promoting a vibrant and joyful existence.

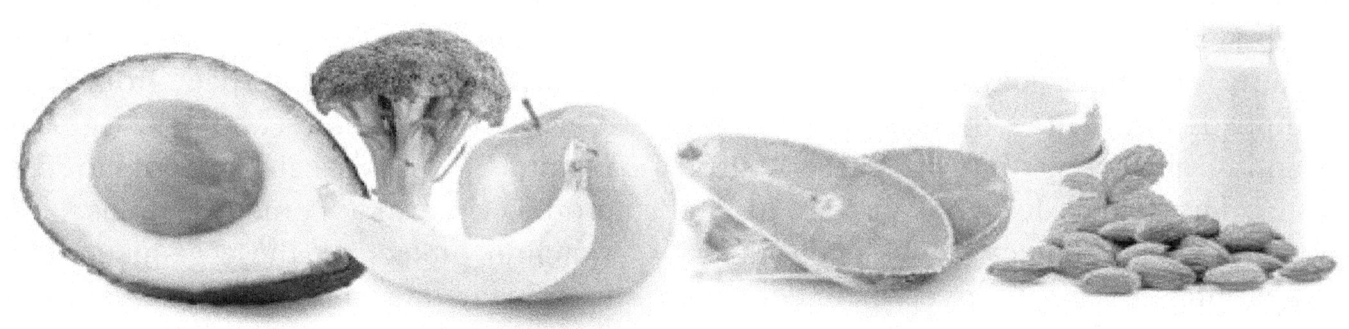

Tailoring a Low Carb Diet to Seniors with Diabetes and Kidney Disease

Seniors with diabetes and renal disease sometimes find themselves at a crossroads in the complex web of health, trying to discover a dietary route that enhances well-being without sacrificing the enjoyment of food. Developing a low-carb diet becomes their compass, helping patients navigate the challenging terrain of controlling chronic diseases while promoting general health.

Recognizing the Intersection: It's important to acknowledge the interaction between diabetes and renal disease in seniors as we explore the complex landscape of these two conditions. Kidney health may be considerably impacted by diabetes, which is defined by decreased insulin function. Long-term high blood sugar levels may be particularly harmful to the kidneys, which are essential for removing waste from the blood. This can result in renal disease. A customized dietary approach that reduces the risks associated with both illnesses is necessary for this delicate tango.

The Low-Carb Advantage: In this complex terrain, a low-carb diet seems to offer a ray of hope. People may better control their blood sugar levels by consuming less carbs, especially processed sugars and starches. This promotes a healthy renal environment by reducing the strain on the kidneys. This nutritional strategy provides seniors with a comprehensive approach to treating the underlying causes of renal disease and diabetes.

Essential Elements of a Senior Low-Carb Diet:

Carbohydrate Quality Over Quantity: Although cutting down on total carbohydrate consumption is important, attention should be paid more attention to the kind of carbs that are ingested. Choose complex, high-fiber foods such as beans, veggies, and whole grains. These give necessary nutrients that are required for general health in addition to stabilizing blood sugar levels.

Moderate Protein Intake: Because too much protein might strain already disabled kidneys, seniors with renal disease may be recommended to consume protein in moderation. Pick lean protein sources like fish, chicken, and plant-based proteins to maintain a balance that supports the function of your muscles without putting too much strain on your kidneys.

Healthy Fats for Satiety: Including foods high in healthy fats, including nuts, avocados, and olive oil, is essential for feeling full and maintaining good health. These fats don't negatively impact blood sugar levels or renal function, but they do add to a fulfilling meal experience.

Consciously Tracking Added Sugar and Salt: Seniors need to watch out for added sugars and salt. Use low-sodium substitutes and natural sweeteners carefully to save your heart and kidneys.

Overcoming Obstacles and Accepting Variability:

Tailored Approaches: Developing a low-carb diet requires a tailored strategy since every senior's health profile is different. Consulting with medical experts, such as doctors and nutritionists, facilitates the creation of a customized strategy that takes into account the unique requirements and difficulties of each person.

Accepting Culinary Creativity: Despite popular belief, a low-carb diet is everything from boring to elderly people. There are many delectable and healthful alternatives available in the wide and diverse food scene. The low-carb palette is a blank canvas just waiting to be explored, so seniors may enjoy every meal to the fullest. Options range from colorful salads to substantial soups.

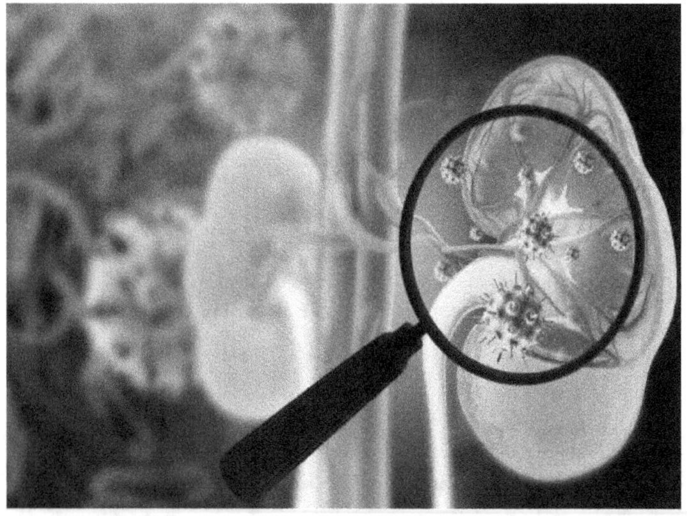

Useful Advice for Execution:

Gradual Transition: Suddenly altering one's diet might be somewhat stressful. It is advised for seniors to gradually switch to a low-carb lifestyle so that their bodies and taste buds have time to adjust.

Frequent Monitoring: It's critical to regularly check kidney function and blood sugar levels. Consultations with medical specialists regularly enable necessary modifications and provide insightful information about how well the low-carb strategy is working.

Including Exercise: Exercise enhances dietary modifications and improves general health. Under the supervision of healthcare professionals, seniors should participate in activities appropriate for their degree of fitness.

Seniors with diabetes and renal illness need a customized low-carb diet that combines scientific principles with humane awareness of their unique requirements. It's a method to take care of these health issues and also enjoy life to the fullest by eating delicious and nutritious food. Let's embrace this journey as well-being advocates, enabling seniors to handle the challenges with resiliency and pleasure.

Chapter 3

NAVIGATING THE RENAL DIET

Overview of a Renal Diet

A renal diet, often referred to as a kidney-friendly diet, is a specific eating schedule created to support kidney function and control the side effects of kidney illness. The goal of this dietary strategy is to restrict the consumption of items that might strain the kidneys while preserving the proper balance of vital nutrients. Whether someone is on dialysis or has just begun kidney illness, maintaining general health greatly depends on following a renal diet.

Important Guidelines for a Renal Diet:

Controlled Protein Intake: Although protein is an essential part of any diet, too much of it may be harmful to kidney disease sufferers. A renal diet entails selecting high-quality protein sources, such as lean meats, fish, poultry, and plant-based proteins, and carefully monitoring protein consumption. This keeps muscle bulk intact without putting too much strain on the kidneys from too much waste.

Monitoring Potassium and Phosphorus Levels: The kidneys control the levels of minerals including potassium and phosphorus. Mineral imbalances may occur in renal disease. To avoid problems including bone and cardiovascular problems, a renal diet limits the consumption of foods rich in phosphorus and potassium, such as dairy products, nuts, and certain fruits and vegetables.

Limitation of Sodium: Sodium, or salt, is important for maintaining fluid balance and controlling blood pressure. Limiting salt consumption is common for people with renal illness to control blood pressure and lessen fluid retention. This entails consuming less processed foods, canned items, and meals that are served at restaurants.

Fluid Management: The body's fluid balance is regulated by the kidneys, and fluid buildup may be problematic in renal disease. A renal diet usually entails limiting the amount of fluid consumed, taking into account foods and drinks that are rich in water content.

<u>Balanced Nutrient Intake:</u> Although controlling certain nutrients is important, a renal diet makes sure that all the necessary nutrients are in balance overall. This involves preserving the proper amounts of vitamins and minerals required for general health, which are often attained by consuming a range of fruits, vegetables, and whole grains.

Adjustment to the Advancement of Illness:

The flexibility of a renal diet to adjust to various stages of kidney disease is a noteworthy feature. In the early stages, modest limitations can be necessary to stop the condition from becoming worse. The food strategy gets increasingly careful as the illness worsens, particularly when dialysis is required, to promote general health and reduce the burden on the kidneys.

Working together with medical professionals:

The implementation of a renal diet requires cooperation from patients, caregivers, and medical experts. When adjusting a diet to suit a patient's demands, dietitians and nutritionists are essential in taking into account the patient's preferences, general health, and renal disease stage.

A renal diet is, in essence, a deliberate and customized approach to maintaining kidney function, controlling symptoms, and improving the quality of life for those who have kidney disease. It goes beyond simple restriction. Those managing the intricacies of renal health may take proactive measures to cultivate their well-being and embrace a lifestyle that meets their particular requirements by choosing their foods with awareness and knowledge.

The kidneys are one of the most important organs in the complex orchestra of bodily activities. These bean-shaped powerhouses are the unsung heroes that toil hard to preserve a delicate equilibrium inside our internal ecology. They are not only quiet filters. A damaged kidney has an impact on the whole body and often interacts with other medical disorders such as diabetes. It is not only a matter of preference; knowing the significance of dietary limitations for renal health is essential to promoting health and delaying the advancement of kidney disease.

We must first make our way across the complex terrain of renal physiology to appreciate the relevance of dietary limitations. The kidneys, which are in charge of eliminating waste and extra fluid from the blood, are especially susceptible to the effects of food decisions. Kidney dysfunction is the result of a delicate balance of electrolytes, minerals, and fluids being upset; this disease is often made worse by diabetes.

The presence of diabetes necessitates a sophisticated strategy in the context of renal health. Diabetes, which is characterized by increased blood glucose levels, directly endangers the kidneys. These organs' complex blood channel network gets damaged, which causes a slow loss of function. This is the point at which dietary limitations become crucial.

Dietary guidelines for kidney health need a careful balancing act, with an emphasis on restricting certain foods to lessen the burden on these essential organs. Among the important participants in this delicate dance are sodium, potassium, and phosphorus. Processed meals often include high levels of salt, which may raise blood pressure and cause fluid retention, which puts more strain on the kidneys. Moderation is necessary to avoid circulatory buildup of potassium, which is essential for nerve and muscle function. Phosphorus control is critical to maintain bone health.

Sodium is a common ingredient in contemporary diets and is often confused with table salt. Its taste-enhancing properties make it appealing, but the damage it does to renal health is too great. One of the main causes of kidney injury is hypertension, which is exacerbated by elevated salt levels. Sodium has a major role in aggravating cardiovascular difficulties for those with diabetes, who already face higher risks of heart disease.

Potassium appears in the complex dance of dietary constraints as a contradiction. Even though it's necessary for body processes, too much of it may seriously harm renal disease patients. Kidney illness, which is often seen in diabetics, may make it difficult for a person to effectively eliminate excess potassium. This imbalance may result in hyperkalemia, a disorder linked to irregular heartbeats, weakening of the muscles, and, in extreme situations, cardiac arrest.

In the context of kidney health, phosphorus—a mineral that is essential for bone health—needs to be carefully considered. Phosphorus levels may rise sharply in renal disease patients, which can lead to bone and mineral abnormalities. Vascular calcification and cardiovascular problems may result from a disruption in the delicate balance between calcium and phosphorus management.

When it comes to food limits for renal health, education is a very useful tool. Knowing the nutritional makeup of food gives people the ability to make decisions that support their health objectives. This understanding affects choices for restaurants and products even beyond the kitchen. Meal planning becomes a deliberate endeavor to support kidney health instead of a tedious chore.

Even if the phrase "dietary restrictions" could make you feel limited, it's important to understand that the goal is deliberate choosing rather than deprivation. Adopting a diet that is healthy for your kidneys allows you to enjoy a wide variety of nutritious meals. Lean meats, nutritious grains, and fresh produce serve as the foundation for a gastronomic tapestry that promotes kidney health and enhances diabetic control.

To sum up, dietary limits are crucial for kidney health because they preserve the delicate balance of our internal ecology, which goes beyond simple food decisions. These limitations serve as a compass for people managing diabetes and renal disease, pointing them in the direction of a life full of energy, resiliency, and empowered well-being.

Keeping elders with diabetes and renal disease in a state of optimal dietary balance is like directing a well-balanced symphony. It requires a sophisticated understanding of how blood sugar control, nutritional decisions, and kidney health interact. We'll examine the fundamentals of a balanced diet designed especially for seniors in this investigation, which provides both nourishment and a route to better health.

Recognizing the Linked Difficulties:

Seniors who have both renal illness and diabetes sometimes find themselves at a dietary crossroads. While renal illness requires a deliberate decrease in specific nutrients to lessen stress on the kidneys, diabetes requires careful management of carbohydrates to maintain blood sugar levels. This delicate tango recognizes the interconnectedness of different health issues and calls for a holistic response.

Mindful Carbohydrate Management: Carbohydrates are essential for controlling blood sugar in elderly diabetics. But not every carbohydrate is made equally. Stable blood sugar regulation may be facilitated by emphasizing complex carbohydrates that have a low glycemic index, such as vegetables, legumes, and whole grains. Equally important is portion management, which enables seniors to partake in a wide range of nutrient-dense meals without experiencing sharp increases in blood sugar.

Strategic Protein Consumption: It is essential to carefully assess protein consumption when renal function declines. Lean protein sources like chicken, fish, tofu, and beans become crucial since high-protein diets may worsen renal stress. Moreover, distributing protein consumption throughout the day delivers the essential amino acids for general health while reducing the burden on the kidneys.

Keeping an eye on Sodium and Phosphorus: Sodium and phosphorus imbalances are a common problem for elderly people with impaired renal function.

Elevated blood pressure and fluid retention may be caused by excess salt, and renal disease may worsen due to excessive phosphorus levels. Seniors may take charge of their nutritional intake by reading product labels to look for hidden nutrients like phosphorus and salt and by selecting fresh, unprocessed meals over processed ones.

Nutrient-Dense, Low Potassium Options: People with renal problems should limit their intake of potassium, a mineral that is essential for many body processes. By including low-potassium fruits and vegetables in their diet, such as green beans, berries, and grapes, seniors may achieve a healthy balance. Boiling and leaching are two cooking techniques that may further lower the potassium level of certain foods, making the menu more varied and appetizing.

Sufficient Hydration: For elderly people with diabetes and renal disease, Sufficient Hydration is a vital component of a balanced diet. Water helps wash waste materials from the kidneys and facilitates digestion and nutritional absorption. Seniors should strive for steady and moderate fluid consumption, making adjustments by their unique health state and any particular advice from medical professionals.

<u>Useful Advice for Execution:</u>

Personalizing Meal Plans: Adapting meal plans to each person's requirements and tastes guarantees that seniors get the right amount of nutrients without feeling constrained. Working with a licensed dietician may provide individualized advice that takes medication, lifestyle, and health conditions into consideration.

Frequent Monitoring: Seniors who have their blood sugar and renal function regularly monitored are better equipped to make educated food decisions. Visiting medical specialists regularly aids in monitoring development and enables essential dietary plan modifications.

Culinary Creativity: Seniors may enjoy a wide variety of tastes while following dietary guidelines by partaking in culinary exploration. Changing up cooking techniques and experimenting with herbs and spices bring flavor to food without sacrificing health objectives.

Seniors with diabetes and renal disease have nutritional demands that must be balanced in a variety of ways, taking into account the complex interplay between food choices and general health. Seniors may start a path toward better health, energy, and a delicious culinary experience by promoting knowledge of the particular obstacles offered by these illnesses and putting practical measures into practice.

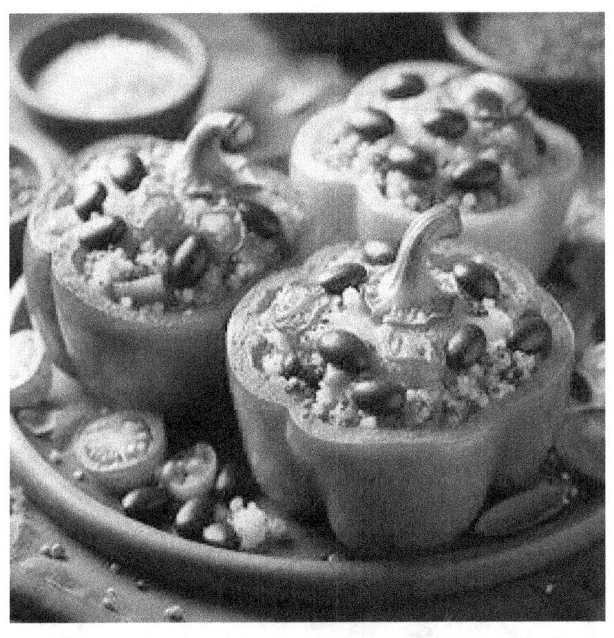

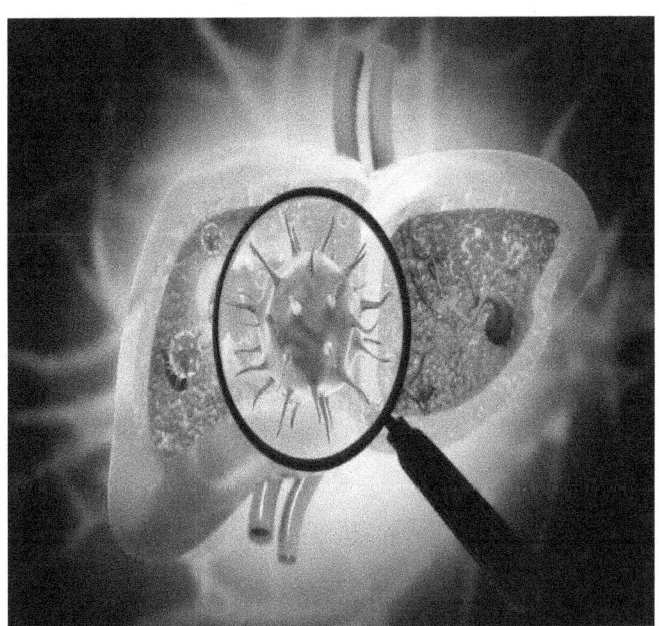

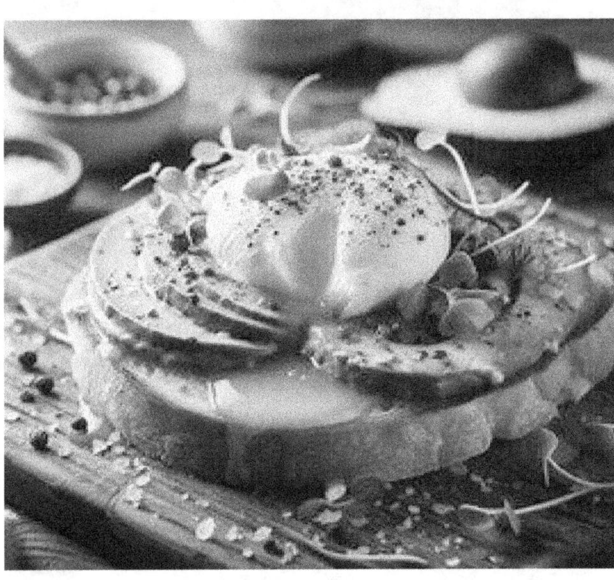

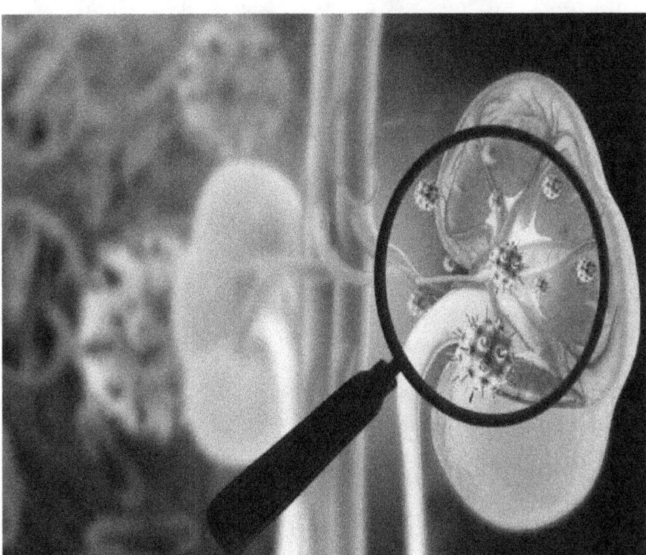

Chapter 4

100+ NOURISHING RECIPES

Breakfast Options

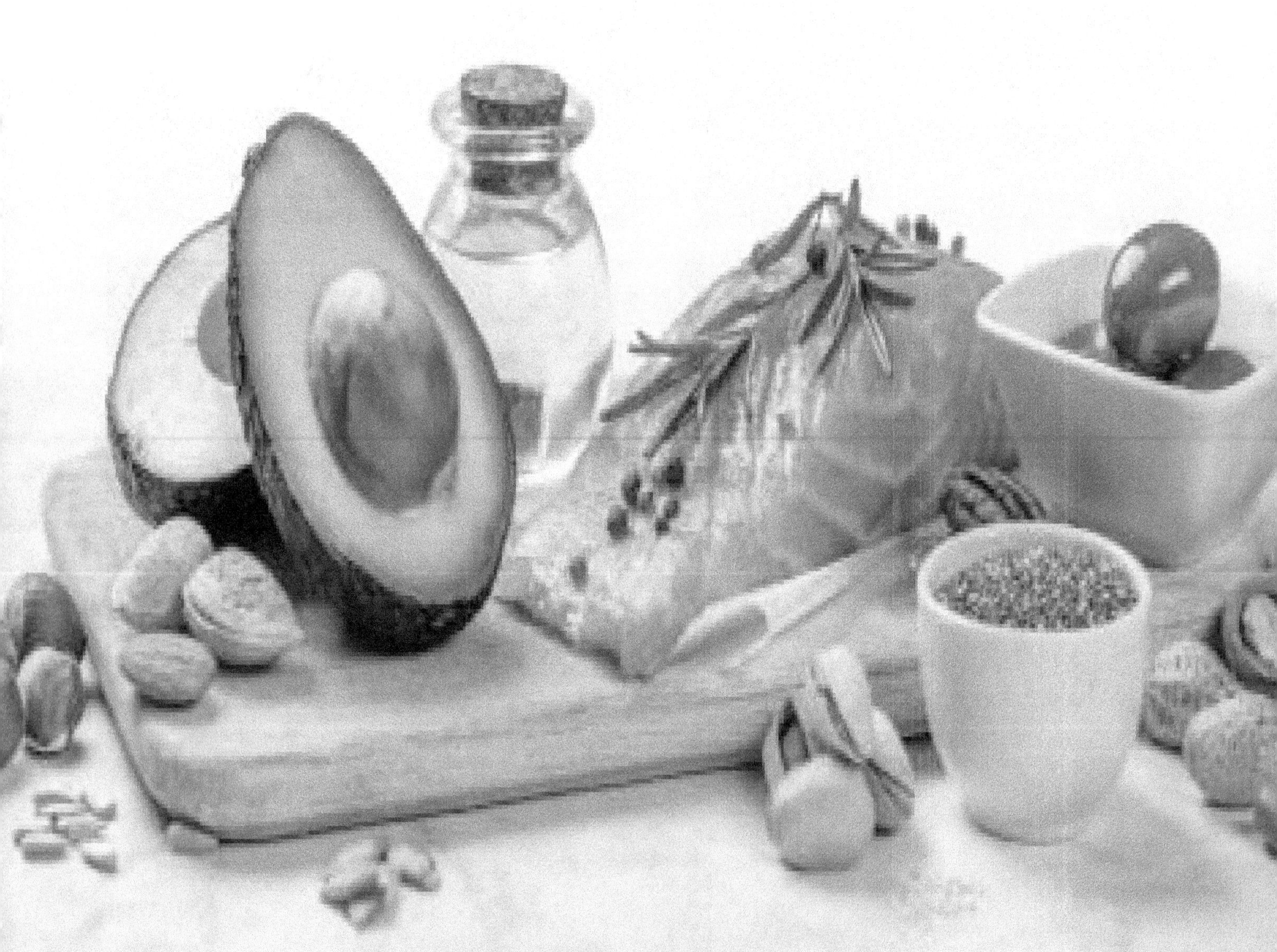

Avocado and Egg Breakfast Bowl

INGREDIENTS

- ❖ 1 ripe avocado
- ❖ 2 eggs
- ❖ 1 tablespoon olive oil
- ❖ Salt and pepper to taste

PREPARATION

- ❖ Cut the avocado in half and scoop out a bit of the flesh to make room for the eggs.
- ❖ Crack an egg into each avocado half.
- ❖ Drizzle with olive oil and season with salt and pepper.
- ❖ Bake in a preheated oven at 375°F (190°C) for 15-20 minutes or until the eggs are cooked to your liking.

Nutrition Information

- ➢ Calories: 320
- ➢ Protein: 12g
- ➢ Carbohydrates: 15g
- ➢ Fiber: 9g
- ➢ Sugars: 1g
- ➢ Total Fat: 25g
- ➢ Cook Time: 15-20 minutes
- ➢ Prep Time: 10 minutes

Greek Yogurt and Berry Parfait

INGREDIENTS

- ❖ 1 cup Greek yogurt
- ❖ 1/2 cup mixed berries (strawberries, blueberries, raspberries)
- ❖ 2 tablespoons chopped nuts (almonds or walnuts)
- ❖ 1 tablespoon honey

PREPARATION

- ❖ In a glass, layer Greek yogurt, mixed berries, and chopped nuts.
- ❖ Drizzle with honey.

Nutrition Information

- ➢ Calories: 250
- ➢ Protein: 18g
- ➢ Carbohydrates: 25g
- ➢ Fiber: 4g
- ➢ Sugars: 18g
- ➢ Total Fat: 10g
- ➢ Cook Time: 5 minutes
- ➢ Prep Time: 5 minutes

Spinach and Feta Omelette

INGREDIENTS

- ❖ 2 eggs
- ❖ 1 cup fresh spinach, chopped
- ❖ 2 tablespoons crumbled feta cheese
- ❖ 1 teaspoon olive oil
- ❖ Salt and pepper to taste

PREPARATION

- ❖ Whisk eggs in a bowl and season with salt and pepper.
- ❖ Heat olive oil in a non-stick pan over medium heat.
- ❖ Add spinach to the pan and cook until wilted.
- ❖ Pour the whisked eggs over the spinach, sprinkle feta on top, and cook until eggs are set.

Nutrition Information

- ➢ Calories: 280
- ➢ Protein: 20g
- ➢ Carbohydrates: 4g
- ➢ Fiber: 2g
- ➢ Sugars: 1g
- ➢ Total Fat: 20g
- ➢ Cook Time: 10 minutes
- ➢ Prep Time: 5 minutes

Chia Seed Pudding with Almond Milk

INGREDIENTS

- ❖ 2 tablespoons chia seeds
- ❖ 1/2 cup unsweetened almond milk
- ❖ 1/4 teaspoon vanilla extract
- ❖ 1/2 cup sliced strawberries

PREPARATION

- ❖ Mix chia seeds, almond milk, and vanilla extract in a bowl.
- ❖ Refrigerate for at least 2 hours or overnight.
- ❖ Top with sliced strawberries before serving.

Nutrition Information

- ➢ Calories: 150
- ➢ Protein: 4g
- ➢ Carbohydrates: 15g
- ➢ Fiber: 9g
- ➢ Sugars: 4g
- ➢ Total Fat: 8g
- ➢ Cook Time: 2 hours (chilling time)
- ➢ Prep Time: 5 minutes

Cottage Cheese and Pineapple Bowl

INGREDIENTS

- ❖ 1/2 cup low-fat cottage cheese
- ❖ 1/2 cup fresh pineapple chunks
- ❖ 1 tablespoon shredded coconut

PREPARATION

- ❖ In a bowl, combine cottage cheese and pineapple chunks.
- ❖ Sprinkle with shredded coconut.

Nutrition Information

- ➢ Calories: 180
- ➢ Protein: 15g
- ➢ Carbohydrates: 20g
- ➢ Fiber: 2g
- ➢ Sugars: 16g
- ➢ Total Fat: 5g
- ➢ Cook Time: 5 minutes
- ➢ Prep Time: 5 minutes

Quinoa Breakfast Bowl

INGREDIENTS

- ❖ 1/2 cup cooked quinoa
- ❖ 1/4 cup unsweetened almond milk
- ❖ 1/2 banana, sliced
- ❖ 1 tablespoon chopped nuts (walnuts or almonds)

PREPARATION

- ❖ In a bowl, combine cooked quinoa and almond milk.
- ❖ Top with sliced banana and chopped nuts.

Nutrition Information

- ➢ Calories: 220
- ➢ Protein: 6g
- ➢ Carbohydrates: 35g
- ➢ Fiber: 4g
- ➢ Sugars: 8g
- ➢ Total Fat: 7g
- ➢ Cook Time: 15 minutes (for quinoa)
- ➢ Prep Time: 5 minutes

Whole Grain Toast with Smashed Avocado and Smoked Salmon

INGREDIENTS

- ❖ 1 slice whole grain bread
- ❖ 1/4 ripe avocado, smashed
- ❖ 2 ounces smoked salmon
- ❖ Lemon juice and black pepper to taste

PREPARATION

- ❖ Toast the whole grain bread.
- ❖ Spread smashed avocado on the toast.
- ❖ Top with smoked salmon, a drizzle of lemon juice, and black pepper.

Nutrition Information

- ➢ Calories: 230
- ➢ Protein: 15g
- ➢ Carbohydrates: 18g
- ➢ Fiber: 5g
- ➢ Sugars: 1g
- ➢ Total Fat: 12g
- ➢ Cook Time: 5 minutes
- ➢ Prep Time: 5 minutes

Blueberry and Almond Smoothie Bowl

INGREDIENTS

- ❖ 1/2 cup blueberries (fresh or frozen)
- ❖ 1/2 banana
- ❖ 1/2 cup unsweetened almond milk
- ❖ 1 tablespoon almond butter
- ❖ 1/4 cup granola

PREPARATION

- ❖ Blend blueberries, banana, almond milk, and almond butter until smooth.
- ❖ Pour into a bowl and top with granola.

Nutrition Information

- ➢ Calories: 280
- ➢ Protein: 8g
- ➢ Carbohydrates: 35g
- ➢ Fiber: 6g
- ➢ Sugars: 15g
- ➢ Total Fat: 12g
- ➢ Cook Time: 5 minutes
- ➢ Prep Time: 5 minutes

Egg and Vegetable Breakfast Wrap

INGREDIENTS

- ❖ 1 whole-grain tortilla
- ❖ 2 eggs, scrambled
- ❖ 1/4 cup diced bell peppers
- ❖ 1/4 cup diced tomatoes
- ❖ 1 tablespoon chopped fresh cilantro

PREPARATION

- ❖ In a skillet, scramble the eggs.
- ❖ Warm the tortilla and fill it with scrambled eggs, bell peppers, tomatoes, and cilantro.

Nutrition Information

- ➢ Calories: 280
- ➢ Protein: 14g
- ➢ Carbohydrates: 25g
- ➢ Fiber: 5g
- ➢ Sugars: 2g
- ➢ Total Fat: 14g
- ➢ Cook Time: 10 minutes
- ➢ Prep Time: 5 minutes

Sweet Potato and Turkey Sausage Hash

INGREDIENTS

- ❖ 1 medium sweet potato, diced
- ❖ 4 ounces lean turkey sausage, crumbled
- ❖ 1/2 onion, chopped
- ❖ 1/2 red bell pepper, chopped
- ❖ 1 tablespoon olive oil
- ❖ Salt and pepper to taste

PREPARATION

- ❖ In a skillet, heat olive oil over medium heat.
- ❖ Add sweet potato, turkey sausage, onion, and red bell pepper. Cook until sweet potatoes are tender and sausage is cooked through.
- ❖ Season with salt and pepper.

Nutrition Information

- ➢ Calories: 320
- ➢ Protein: 15g
- ➢ Carbohydrates: 30g
- ➢ Fiber: 5g
- ➢ Sugars: 8g
- ➢ Total Fat: 16g
- ➢ Cook Time: 20 minutes
- ➢ Prep Time: 10 minutes

Grilled Lemon Herb Salmon

INGREDIENTS

* 4 salmon fillets
* 2 tablespoons olive oil
* 1 tablespoon fresh lemon juice
* 1 teaspoon dried thyme
* Salt and pepper to taste

PREPARATION

* Preheat the grill to medium-high heat.
* In a small bowl, mix olive oil, lemon juice, thyme, salt, and pepper.
* Brush the salmon fillets with the mixture.
* Grill the salmon for 4-5 minutes per side or until cooked through.
* Serve hot.

Nutrition Information

* Calories: 250
* Protein: 30g
* Fat: 14g
* Carbohydrates: 1g
* Fiber: 0.5g
* Cook Time: 10 minutes
* Prep Time: 10 minutes

Zucchini Noodles with Pesto Chicken

INGREDIENTS

* 2 medium zucchinis, spiralized
* 1 lb chicken breast, cooked and shredded
* ½ cup cherry tomatoes, halved
* ¼ cup basil pesto
* Salt and pepper to taste

PREPARATION

* Saute spiralized zucchini in a pan until tender.
* In a bowl, mix zucchini, shredded chicken, cherry tomatoes, and pesto.
* Season with salt and pepper.
* Toss gently until well combined.
* Serve warm.

Nutrition Information

* Calories: 280
* Protein: 35g
* Fat: 10g
* Carbohydrates: 8g
* Fiber: 3g
* Cook Time: 15 minutes
* Prep Time: 15 minutes

Cucumber and Avocado Salad

INGREDIENTS

- ❖ 2 cucumbers, sliced
- ❖ 1 avocado, diced
- ❖ 1 cup cherry tomatoes, halved
- ❖ ¼ cup red onion, thinly sliced
- ❖ 2 tablespoons olive oil
- ❖ 1 tablespoon balsamic vinegar
- ❖ Salt and pepper to taste

PREPARATION

- ❖ In a large bowl, combine cucumbers, avocado, cherry tomatoes, and red onion.
- ❖ Drizzle olive oil and balsamic vinegar over the salad.
- ❖ Season with salt and pepper.
- ❖ Toss gently to coat.
- ❖ Refrigerate before serving.

Nutrition Information

- ➢ Calories: 180
- ➢ Protein: 3g
- ➢ Fat: 14g
- ➢ Carbohydrates: 15g
- ➢ Fiber: 6g
- ➢ Cook Time: 10 minutes
- ➢ Prep Time: 15 minutes

Turkey and Vegetable Stir-Fry

INGREDIENTS

- ❖ 1 lb turkey breast, thinly sliced
- ❖ 2 cups broccoli florets
- ❖ 1 bell pepper, sliced
- ❖ 1 cup snap peas
- ❖ 2 tablespoons low-sodium soy sauce
- ❖ 1 tablespoon sesame oil
- ❖ 1 teaspoon ginger, minced
- ❖ 2 cloves garlic, minced

PREPARATION

- ❖ Heat sesame oil in a wok or skillet over medium-high heat.
- ❖ Add turkey slices and stir-fry until cooked.
- ❖ Add broccoli, bell pepper, and snap peas. Continue to stir-fry until vegetables are tender-crisp.
- ❖ Mix in soy sauce, ginger, and garlic.
- ❖ Cook for an additional 2-3 minutes, stirring continuously.
- ❖ Serve hot.

Nutrition Information

- ➢ Calories: 280
- ➢ Protein: 35g
- ➢ Fat: 8g
- ➢ Carbohydrates: 15g
- ➢ Fiber: 5g
- ➢ Cook Time: 20 minutes
- ➢ Prep Time: 15 minutes

Cauliflower Rice with Shrimp

INGREDIENTS

- ❖ 1 lb shrimp, peeled and deveined
- ❖ 4 cups cauliflower rice
- ❖ 1 cup bell peppers, diced
- ❖ 2 tablespoons olive oil
- ❖ 1 teaspoon cumin
- ❖ ½ teaspoon paprika
- ❖ Salt and pepper to taste

PREPARATION

- ❖ In a large skillet, heat olive oil over medium heat.
- ❖ Add shrimp and cook until pink.
- ❖ Stir in cauliflower rice, bell peppers, cumin, paprika, salt, and pepper.
- ❖ Cook for 5-7 minutes until cauliflower rice is tender.
- ❖ Serve warm.

Nutrition Information

- ➢ Calories: 220
- ➢ Protein: 25g
- ➢ Fat: 10g
- ➢ Carbohydrates: 8g
- ➢ Fiber: 4g
- ➢ Cook Time: 15 minutes
- ➢ Prep Time: 10 minutes

Spinach and Feta Stuffed Chicken Breast

INGREDIENTS

- ❖ 4 chicken breasts
- ❖ 2 cups fresh spinach, chopped
- ❖ ½ cup feta cheese, crumbled
- ❖ 1 teaspoon garlic powder
- ❖ Salt and pepper to taste

PREPARATION

- ❖ Preheat the oven to 375°F (190°C).
- ❖ In a bowl, mix chopped spinach, feta, garlic powder, salt, and pepper.
- ❖ Cut a pocket in each chicken breast and stuff with the spinach-feta mixture.
- ❖ Place the stuffed chicken breasts in a baking dish.
- ❖ Bake for 25-30 minutes or until chicken is cooked through.
- ❖ Serve hot.

Nutrition Information

- ➢ Calories: 280
- ➢ Protein: 35g
- ➢ Fat: 12g
- ➢ Carbohydrates: 3g
- ➢ Fiber: 1.5g
- ➢ Cook Time: 30 minutes
- ➢ Prep Time: 15 minutes

Eggplant and Tomato Bake

INGREDIENTS

* 2 medium-sized eggplants, sliced
* 2 cups cherry tomatoes, halved
* 1 cup mozzarella cheese, shredded
* 2 tablespoons olive oil
* 2 teaspoons Italian seasoning
* Salt and pepper to taste

PREPARATION

* Preheat the oven to 400°F (200°C).
* Arrange eggplant slices on a baking sheet and brush with olive oil.
* Sprinkle with Italian seasoning, salt, and pepper.
* Bake for 15-20 minutes until eggplant is tender.
* In a separate bowl, combine cherry tomatoes and mozzarella.
* Place the tomato and cheese mixture on top of the baked eggplant.
* Broil for an additional 5 minutes until cheese is melted and bubbly.
* Serve warm.

Nutrition Information

* Calories: 220
* Protein: 10g
* Fat: 15g
* Carbohydrates: 15g
* Fiber: 7g
* Cook Time: 25 minutes
* Prep Time: 15 minutes

Avocado and Tuna Salad

INGREDIENTS

* 2 cans tuna, drained
* 2 avocados, diced
* 1 cucumber, diced
* 1/4 cup red onion, finely chopped
* 2 tablespoons olive oil
* 1 tablespoon lemon juice
* Salt and pepper to taste

PREPARATION

* In a bowl, combine tuna, avocados, cucumber, and red onion.
* Drizzle with olive oil and lemon juice.
* Season with salt and pepper.
* Gently toss until ingredients are well mixed.
* Refrigerate for 30 minutes before serving.

Nutrition Information

* Calories: 300
* Protein: 25g
* Fat: 20g
* Carbohydrates: 10g
* Fiber: 7g
* Cook Time: 10 minutes
* Prep Time: 15 minutes

Greek Yogurt Parfait

INGREDIENTS

- ❖ In a glass or bowl, layer Greek yogurt, blueberries, and strawberries.
- ❖ Repeat the layers until the container is filled.
- ❖ Top with chopped nuts and drizzle with honey.
- ❖ Serve chilled.

PREPARATION

- ❖ In a glass or bowl, layer Greek yogurt, blueberries, and strawberries.
- ❖ Repeat the layers until the container is filled.
- ❖ Top with chopped nuts and drizzle with honey.
- ❖ Serve chilled.

Nutrition Information

- ➢ Calories: 220
- ➢ Protein: 15g
- ➢ Fat: 10g
- ➢ Carbohydrates: 20g
- ➢ Fiber: 3g
- ➢ Cook Time: 5 minutes
- ➢ Prep Time: 10 minutes

Berry Almond Chia Pudding

INGREDIENTS

- ❖ 1/4 cup chia seeds
- ❖ 1 cup almond milk
- ❖ 1/2 teaspoon vanilla extract
- ❖ 1/2 cup mixed berries (blueberries, raspberries, strawberries)
- ❖ 2 tablespoons sliced almonds

PREPARATION

- ❖ In a bowl, mix chia seeds, almond milk, and vanilla extract.
- ❖ Let the mixture sit for 15-20 minutes or until it thickens.
- ❖ Layer chia pudding with mixed berries in serving glasses.
- ❖ Top with sliced almonds.
- ❖ Refrigerate for at least 2 hours before serving.

Nutrition Information

- ➢ Calories: 180
- ➢ Protein: 5g
- ➢ Fat: 10g
- ➢ Carbohydrates: 20g
- ➢ Fiber: 8g
- ➢ Cook Time: 5 minutes
- ➢ Prep Time: 15 minutes

Grilled Salmon Salad with Lemon Vinaigrette

INGREDIENTS

- ❖ 6 oz salmon fillet
- ❖ Mixed salad greens
- ❖ Cherry tomatoes, halved
- ❖ Cucumber, sliced
- ❖ Red onion, thinly sliced
- ❖ Olive oil, lemon juice, Dijon mustard, salt, and pepper for vinaigrette

PREPARATION

- ❖ Grill salmon until cooked.
- ❖ Mix salad greens, tomatoes, cucumber, and red onion.
- ❖ Whisk together olive oil, lemon juice, Dijon mustard, salt, and pepper for dressing.
- ❖ Flake salmon over the salad and drizzle with vinaigrette.

Nutrition Information

- ➢ Calories: 320
- ➢ Protein: 25g
- ➢ Carbohydrates: 10g
- ➢ Fat: 20g
- ➢ Cook Time: 10 minutes
- ➢ Prep Time: 15 minutes

Chicken and Vegetable Stir-Fry

INGREDIENTS

- ❖ 1 cup chicken breast, sliced
- ❖ Broccoli florets
- ❖ Bell peppers, sliced
- ❖ Snap peas
- ❖ Garlic, minced
- ❖ Low-sodium soy sauce

PREPARATION

- ❖ Stir-fry chicken until cooked.
- ❖ Add vegetables and garlic, stir-frying until tender.
- ❖ Drizzle with low-sodium soy sauce.

Nutrition Information

- ➢ Calories: 280
- ➢ Protein: 30g
- ➢ Carbohydrates: 12g
- ➢ Fat: 12g
- ➢ Cook Time: 15 minutes
- ➢ Prep Time: 20 minutes

Quinoa and Black Bean Bowl

INGREDIENTS

- 1 cup cooked quinoa
- Black beans, drained and rinsed
- Avocado, diced
- Cherry tomatoes, halved
- Cilantro, chopped
- Lime juice, salt, and pepper

PREPARATION

- Mix quinoa, black beans, avocado, and tomatoes.
- Sprinkle with cilantro and drizzle with lime juice.
- Season with salt and pepper to taste.

Nutrition Information

- Calories: 320
- Protein: 15g
- Carbohydrates: 45g
- Fat: 10g
- Cook Time: 20 minutes
- Prep Time: 10 minutes

Mushroom and Spinach Omelette

INGREDIENTS

- 2 eggs
- Mushrooms, sliced
- Fresh spinach leaves
- Feta cheese, crumbled
- Olive oil
- Salt and pepper

PREPARATION

- Sauté mushrooms in olive oil until tender.
- Add fresh spinach and cook until wilted.
- Whisk eggs, pour over the vegetables, and sprinkle with feta.
- Cook until the eggs are set, then fold the omelette.

Nutrition Information

- Calories: 280
- Protein: 18g
- Carbohydrates: 6g
- Fat: 20g
- Cook Time: 10 minutes
- Prep Time: 15 minutes

Turkey and Vegetable Skewers

INGREDIENTS

- ❖ Turkey breast, cut into cubes
- ❖ Zucchini, sliced
- ❖ Cherry tomatoes
- ❖ Red onion, diced
- ❖ Olive oil, garlic powder, paprika, salt, and pepper

PREPARATION

- ❖ Thread turkey, zucchini, tomatoes, and onion onto skewers.
- ❖ Mix olive oil, garlic powder, paprika, salt, and pepper.
- ❖ Brush the skewers with the mixture and grill until turkey is cooked.

Nutrition Information

- ➢ Calories: 250
- ➢ Protein: 28g
- ➢ Carbohydrates: 10g
- ➢ Fat: 10g
- ➢ Cook Time: 15 minutes
- ➢ Prep Time: 20 minutes

Spinach and Lentil Soup

INGREDIENTS

- ❖ 1 cup lentils, rinsed
- ❖ Spinach, chopped
- ❖ Carrots, diced
- ❖ Celery, chopped
- ❖ Garlic, minced
- ❖ Low-sodium vegetable broth, cumin, coriander, salt, and pepper

PREPARATION

- ❖ Sauté garlic, add lentils, carrots, and celery.
- ❖ Pour in vegetable broth, season with cumin, coriander, salt, and pepper.
- ❖ Simmer until lentils are tender, then stir in chopped spinach.

Nutrition Information

- ➢ Calories: 220
- ➢ Protein: 15g
- ➢ Carbohydrates: 40g
- ➢ Fat: 2g
- ➢ Cook Time: 30 minutes
- ➢ Prep Time: 15 minutes

Salmon and Asparagus Foil Pack

INGREDIENTS

- ❖ 6 oz salmon fillet
- ❖ Asparagus spears
- ❖ Lemon slices
- ❖ Dill, chopped
- ❖ Olive oil, salt, and pepper

PREPARATION

- ❖ Place salmon on a foil sheet, surround with asparagus.
- ❖ Drizzle with olive oil, sprinkle with dill, salt, and pepper.
- ❖ Seal the foil pack and bake until salmon is cooked through.

Nutrition Information

- ➢ Calories: 280
- ➢ Protein: 25g
- ➢ Carbohydrates: 10g
- ➢ Fat: 16g
- ➢ Cook Time: 20 minutes
- ➢ Prep Time: 10 minutes

Eggplant and Tomato Bake

INGREDIENTS

- ❖ Eggplant, sliced
- ❖ Tomatoes, sliced
- ❖ Mozzarella cheese, shredded
- ❖ Fresh basil leaves
- ❖ Olive oil, balsamic glaze, salt, and pepper

PREPARATION

- ❖ Layer eggplant and tomato slices in a baking dish.
- ❖ Drizzle with olive oil, season with salt and pepper.
- ❖ Top with mozzarella and bake until cheese is melted.
- ❖ Garnish with fresh basil and drizzle with balsamic glaze

Nutrition Information

- ➢ Calories: 230
- ➢ Protein: 12g
- ➢ Carbohydrates: 15g
- ➢ Fat: 15g
- ➢ Cook Time: 25 minutes
- ➢ Prep Time: 15 minutes

Cauliflower and Chickpea Curry

INGREDIENTS

- ❖ Cauliflower florets
- ❖ Chickpeas, drained and rinsed
- ❖ Onion, diced
- ❖ Coconut milk
- ❖ Curry powder, turmeric, garlic powder, salt, and pepper

PREPARATION

- ❖ Sauté onions, add cauliflower, chickpeas, and spices.
- ❖ Pour in coconut milk and simmer until cauliflower is tender.

Nutrition Information

- ➢ Calories: 260
- ➢ Protein: 14g
- ➢ Carbohydrates: 30g
- ➢ Fat: 10g
- ➢ Cook Time: 25 minutes
- ➢
- ➢ Prep Time: 15 minutes

Greek Chicken Wrap

INGREDIENTS

- ❖ Grilled chicken breast, sliced
- ❖ Whole-grain wrap
- ❖ Tzatziki sauce
- ❖ Cherry tomatoes, sliced
- ❖ Cucumber, julienned
- ❖ Feta cheese, crumbled
- ❖ Fresh dill

PREPARATION

- ❖ Spread tzatziki on the wrap, layer with chicken, tomatoes, cucumber, feta, and fresh dill.
- ❖ Fold the sides and roll into a wrap.

Nutrition Information

- ➢ Calories: 310
- ➢ Protein: 25g
- ➢ Carbohydrates: 20g
- ➢ Fat: 15g
- ➢ Cook Time: 15 minutes
- ➢ Prep Time: 10 minutes

Grilled Lemon Herb Salmon

INGREDIENTS

- ❖ 4 salmon fillets
- ❖ 2 tablespoons olive oil
- ❖ 1 lemon (zested and juiced)
- ❖ 2 cloves garlic (minced)
- ❖ 1 teaspoon dried dill
- ❖ Salt and pepper to taste

PREPARATION

- ❖ In a bowl, mix olive oil, lemon zest, lemon juice, minced garlic, dill, salt, and pepper.
- ❖ Marinate salmon fillets in the mixture for 30 minutes.
- ❖ Preheat grill and cook salmon for 4-5 minutes per side or until flaky.
- ❖ Serve with a side of steamed vegetables.

Nutrition Information

- Calories: 300
- ➢ Protein: 25g
- ➢ Carbohydrates: 2g
- ➢ Fat: 20g
- ➢ Fiber: 1g
- ➢ Cook Time: 10 minutes
- ➢ Prep Time: 40 minutes

Chicken and Vegetable Stir-Fry

INGREDIENTS

- ❖ 1 lb boneless, skinless chicken breast (sliced)
- ❖ 2 cups broccoli florets
- ❖ 1 bell pepper (sliced)
- ❖ 1 cup snap peas
- ❖ 2 tablespoons low-sodium soy sauce
- ❖ 1 tablespoon olive oil
- ❖ 1 teaspoon ginger (minced)
- ❖ 2 cloves garlic (minced)

PREPARATION

- ❖ Heat olive oil in a wok or skillet, add chicken and cook until browned.
- ❖ Add ginger and garlic, stir-fry for 1-2 minutes.
- ❖ Add broccoli, bell pepper, and snap peas, cook until vegetables are tender.
- ❖ Stir in soy sauce and cook for an additional 2 minutes.

Nutrition Information

- ➢ Calories: 250
- ➢ Protein: 30g
- ➢ Carbohydrates: 10g
- ➢ Fat: 8g
- ➢ Fiber: 4g
- ➢ Cook Time: 15 minutes
- ➢ Prep Time: 20 minutes

Turkey and Quinoa Stuffed Peppers

INGREDIENTS

- ❖ 4 large bell peppers (halved)
- ❖ 1 lb ground turkey
- ❖ 1 cup cooked quinoa
- ❖ 1 can black beans (drained and rinsed)
- ❖ 1 cup salsa
- ❖ 1 teaspoon cumin
- ❖ 1 teaspoon chili powder

PREPARATION

- ❖ Preheat oven to 375°F (190°C).
- ❖ Brown turkey in a pan, add cooked quinoa, black beans, salsa, cumin, and chili powder.
- ❖ Stuff bell peppers with the turkey mixture.
- ❖ Bake for 25-30 minutes until peppers are tender.

Nutrition Information

- ➢ Calories: 320
- ➢ Protein: 25g
- ➢ Carbohydrates: 30g
- ➢ Fat: 10g
- ➢ Fiber: 8g
- ➢ Cook Time: 30 minutes
- ➢ Prep Time: 25 minutes

Baked Lemon Herb Chicken Thighs

INGREDIENTS

- ❖ 4 chicken thighs (bone-in, skin-on)
- ❖ 2 tablespoons olive oil
- ❖ 1 lemon (zested and juiced)
- ❖ 2 teaspoons dried thyme
- ❖ 1 teaspoon garlic powder
- ❖ Salt and pepper to taste

PREPARATION

- ❖ Preheat the oven to 400°F (200°C).
- ❖ In a bowl, combine olive oil, lemon zest, lemon juice, thyme, garlic powder, salt, and pepper.
- ❖ Place chicken thighs in a baking dish and coat with the lemon herb mixture.
- ❖ Bake for 35-40 minutes or until chicken reaches an internal temperature of 165°F (74°C).

Nutrition Information

- ➢ Calories: 280
- ➢ Protein: 22g
- ➢ Carbohydrates: 1g
- ➢ Fat: 20g
- ➢ Fiber: 0g
- ➢ Cook Time: 40 minutes
- ➢ Prep Time: 10 minutes

Vegetable and Lentil Soup

INGREDIENTS

- ❖ 1 cup green or brown lentils (rinsed)
- ❖ 1 onion (chopped)
- ❖ 2 carrots (chopped)
- ❖ 2 celery stalks (chopped)
- ❖ 3 cloves garlic (minced)
- ❖ 6 cups low-sodium vegetable broth
- ❖ 1 teaspoon cumin
- ❖ 1 teaspoon paprika
- ❖ Salt and pepper to taste

PREPARATION

- ❖ In a large pot, sauté onion, carrots, celery, and garlic until softened.
- ❖ Add lentils, vegetable broth, cumin, paprika, salt, and pepper.
- ❖ Simmer for 25-30 minutes until lentils are tender.

Nutrition Information

- ➤ Calories: 220
- ➤ Protein: 14g
- ➤ Carbohydrates: 38g
- ➤ Fat: 1g
- ➤ Fiber: 16g
- ➤ Cook Time: 30 minutes
- ➤ Prep Time: 15 minutes

Shrimp and Zucchini Noodles Stir-Fry

INGREDIENTS

- ❖ 1 lb shrimp (peeled and deveined)
- ❖ 4 medium zucchinis (spiralized)
- ❖ 1 bell pepper (sliced)
- ❖ 2 tablespoons low-sodium soy sauce
- ❖ 1 tablespoon sesame oil
- ❖ 1 teaspoon ginger (minced)
- ❖ 2 cloves garlic (minced)

PREPARATION

- ❖ In a wok or skillet, sauté shrimp until pink.
- ❖ Add ginger and garlic, stir-fry for 1-2 minutes.
- ❖ Add zucchini noodles and bell pepper, cook until vegetables are tender.
- ❖ Stir in soy sauce and sesame oil, cook for an additional 2 minutes.

Nutrition Information

- ➤ Calories: 180
- ➤ Protein: 20g
- ➤ Carbohydrates: 10g
- ➤ Fat: 7g
- ➤ Fiber: 3g
- ➤ Cook Time: 15 minutes
- ➤ Prep Time: 20 minutes

Quinoa and Vegetable Stuffed Acorn Squash

INGREDIENTS

- ❖ 2 acorn squash (halved and seeded)
- ❖ 1 cup cooked quinoa
- ❖ 1 cup cherry tomatoes (halved)
- ❖ 1 cup spinach (chopped)
- ❖ 1/2 cup feta cheese (crumbled)
- ❖ 2 tablespoons balsamic glaze

PREPARATION

- ❖ Preheat oven to 400°F (200°C).
- ❖ Roast acorn squash halves for 30 minutes.
- ❖ In a bowl, mix cooked quinoa, cherry tomatoes, spinach, and feta.
- ❖ Stuff each squash half with the quinoa mixture and drizzle with balsamic glaze.

Nutrition Information

- ➢ Calories: 280
- ➢ Protein: 9g
- ➢ Carbohydrates: 50g
- ➢ Fat: 6g
- ➢ Fiber: 8g
- ➢ Cook Time: 30 minutes
- ➢ Prep Time: 20 minutes

Lemon Garlic Baked Cod

INGREDIENTS

- ❖ 4 cod fillets
- ❖ 3 tablespoons olive oil
- ❖ 2 lemons (zested and juiced)
- ❖ 3 cloves garlic (minced)
- ❖ 1 teaspoon dried oregano
- ❖ Salt and pepper to taste

PREPARATION

- ❖ Preheat the oven to 375°F (190°C).
- ❖ Place cod fillets in a baking dish.
- ❖ In a bowl, combine olive oil, lemon zest, lemon juice, minced garlic, oregano, salt, and pepper.
- ❖ Pour the mixture over the cod and bake for 20-25 minutes or until fish flakes easily.

Nutrition Information

- ➢ Calories: 220
- ➢ Protein: 25g
- ➢ Carbohydrates: 3g
- ➢ Fat: 12g
- ➢ Fiber: 1g
- ➢ Cook Time: 25 minutes
- ➢ Prep Time: 15 minutes

Spinach and Feta Stuffed Chicken Breast

INGREDIENTS

- ❖ 4 boneless, skinless chicken breasts
- ❖ 1 cup fresh spinach (chopped)
- ❖ 1/2 cup feta cheese (crumbled)
- ❖ 2 tablespoons olive oil
- ❖ 1 teaspoon dried basil
- ❖ Salt and pepper to taste

PREPARATION

- ❖ Preheat the oven to 400°F (200°C).
- ❖ Butterfly each chicken breast.
- ❖ In a bowl, mix chopped spinach, feta, olive oil, dried basil, salt, and pepper.
- ❖ Stuff each chicken breast with the spinach and feta mixture, then bake for 25-30 minutes.

Nutrition Information

- ➢ Calories: 280
- ➢ Protein: 30g
- ➢ Carbohydrates: 2g
- ➢ Fat: 16g
- ➢ Fiber: 1g
- ➢ Cook Time: 30 minutes
- ➢ Prep Time: 20 minutes

Mediterranean Chickpea Salad

INGREDIENTS

- ❖ 2 cans chickpeas (drained and rinsed)
- ❖ 1 cucumber (diced)
- ❖ 1 cup cherry tomatoes (halved)
- ❖ 1/2 red onion (finely chopped)
- ❖ 1/2 cup Kalamata olives (sliced)
- ❖ 1/4 cup feta cheese (crumbled)
- ❖ 3 tablespoons olive oil
- ❖ 2 tablespoons red wine vinegar
- ❖ 1 teaspoon dried oregano
- ❖ Salt and pepper to taste

PREPARATION

- ❖ In a large bowl, combine chickpeas, cucumber, cherry tomatoes, red onion, olives, and feta.
- ❖ In a small bowl, whisk together olive oil, red wine vinegar, dried oregano, salt, and pepper.
- ❖ Pour the dressing over the salad and toss gently.

Nutrition Information

- ➢ Calories: 320
- ➢ Protein: 12g
- ➢ Carbohydrates: 35g
- ➢ Fat: 16g
- ➢ Fiber: 10g
- ➢ Prep Time: 15 minutes

Grilled Salmon with Lemon Herb Glaze

INGREDIENTS

- 4 salmon fillets
- 2 tablespoons olive oil
- 1 lemon (zested and juiced)
- 2 cloves garlic (minced)
- 1 teaspoon dried oregano
- Salt and pepper to taste

PREPARATION

- Preheat grill to medium-high heat.
- In a bowl, mix olive oil, lemon zest, lemon juice, minced garlic, dried oregano, salt, and pepper.
- Brush the salmon fillets with the lemon herb mixture.
- Grill salmon for 4-5 minutes per side or until cooked through.
- Serve hot and garnish with additional lemon slices.

Nutrition Information

- Calories: 300
- Protein: 28g
- Carbohydrates: 2g
- Fat: 20g
- Fiber: 1g
- Cook Time: 10 minutes
- Prep Time: 15 minutes

Turkey and Vegetable Stir-Fry

INGREDIENTS

- 1 lb lean ground turkey
- 2 cups broccoli florets
- 1 bell pepper (sliced)
- 1 cup snap peas
- 3 tablespoons low-sodium soy sauce
- 2 tablespoons olive oil
- 1 teaspoon ginger (grated)
- 2 cloves garlic (minced)

PREPARATION

- In a large skillet, heat olive oil over medium-high heat.
- Add ground turkey and cook until browned.
- Add ginger and garlic, stir for 1 minute.
- Add broccoli, bell pepper, and snap peas. Stir-fry until vegetables are tender.
- Pour soy sauce over the mixture and stir well.
- Serve over cauliflower rice or whole-grain rice.

Nutrition Information

- Calories: 320
- Protein: 25g
- Carbohydrates: 12g
- Fat: 18g
- Fiber: 4g
- Cook Time: 20 minutes
- Prep Time: 15 minutes

Chicken and Vegetable Quinoa Bowl

INGREDIENTS

- ❖ 1 lb chicken breast (cubed)
- ❖ 1 cup quinoa (cooked)
- ❖ 1 zucchini (sliced)
- ❖ 1 cup cherry tomatoes (halved)
- ❖ 1/4 cup feta cheese (crumbled)
- ❖ 2 tablespoons balsamic vinaigrette
- ❖ 1 tablespoon olive oil
- ❖ Salt and pepper to taste

PREPARATION

- ❖ Season chicken cubes with salt and pepper.
- ❖ In a skillet, heat olive oil over medium heat. Cook chicken until no longer pink.
- ❖ In a bowl, combine cooked quinoa, zucchini, cherry tomatoes, and cooked chicken.
- ❖ Drizzle balsamic vinaigrette over the mixture and toss.
- ❖ Top with crumbled feta cheese before serving.

Nutrition Information

- ➢ Calories: 380
- ➢ Protein: 30g
- ➢ Carbohydrates: 30g
- ➢ Fat: 15g
- ➢ Fiber: 5g
- ➢ Cook Time: 25 minutes
- ➢ Prep Time: 15 minutes

Lentil and Vegetable Stew

INGREDIENTS

- ❖ 1 cup dry green lentils (rinsed)
- ❖ 1 onion (chopped)
- ❖ 2 carrots (sliced)
- ❖ 2 celery stalks (chopped)
- ❖ 3 cloves garlic (minced)
- ❖ 1 can (14 oz) diced tomatoes
- ❖ 4 cups vegetable broth
- ❖ 1 teaspoon cumin
- ❖ 1 teaspoon smoked paprika
- ❖ Salt and pepper to taste

PREPARATION

- ❖ In a large pot, sauté onions, carrots, celery, and garlic until softened.
- ❖ Add lentils, diced tomatoes, vegetable broth, cumin, smoked paprika, salt, and pepper.
- ❖ Bring to a boil, then reduce heat and simmer for 25-30 minutes or until lentils are tender.
- ❖ Adjust seasoning if necessary before serving.

Nutrition Information

- ➢ Calories: 280
- ➢ Protein: 18g
- ➢ Carbohydrates: 45g
- ➢ Fat: 2g
- ➢ Fiber: 18g
- ➢ Cook Time: 35 minutes
- ➢ Prep Time: 15 minutes

Baked Cod with Roasted Vegetables

INGREDIENTS

- ❖ 4 cod fillets
- ❖ 2 cups mixed vegetables (bell peppers, cherry tomatoes, zucchini)
- ❖ 2 tablespoons olive oil
- ❖ 1 teaspoon dried thyme
- ❖ 1 teaspoon garlic powder
- ❖ Lemon wedges for serving
- ❖ Salt and pepper to taste

PREPARATION

- ❖ Preheat oven to 400°F (200°C).
- ❖ Place cod fillets on a baking sheet and surround them with mixed vegetables.
- ❖ Drizzle olive oil over the fish and vegetables. Sprinkle dried thyme, garlic powder, salt, and pepper.
- ❖ Bake for 20-25 minutes or until the fish flakes easily with a fork.
- ❖ Serve with a squeeze of lemon.

Nutrition Information

- ➢ Calories: 250
- ➢ Protein: 30g
- ➢ Carbohydrates: 10g
- ➢ Fat: 10g
- ➢ Fiber: 3g
- ➢ Cook Time: 25 minutes
- ➢ Prep Time: 15 minutes

Shrimp and Asparagus Stir-Fry

INGREDIENTS

- ❖ 1 lb shrimp (peeled and deveined)
- ❖ 1 bunch asparagus (trimmed and cut into pieces)
- ❖ 1 red onion (sliced)
- ❖ 3 tablespoons low-sodium soy sauce
- ❖ 2 tablespoons sesame oil
- ❖ 1 tablespoon honey
- ❖ 2 teaspoons cornstarch
- ❖ 1 teaspoon ginger (minced)
- ❖ 2 cloves garlic (minced)

PREPARATION

- ❖ In a small bowl, mix soy sauce, sesame oil, honey, and cornstarch. Set aside.
- ❖ In a wok or skillet, stir-fry shrimp until pink. Remove and set aside.
- ❖ Stir-fry asparagus and red onion until tender-crisp.
- ❖ Add minced ginger and garlic, stir for 1 minute.
- ❖ Return shrimp to the pan, pour the sauce over, and toss until coated.
- ❖ Serve over cauliflower rice.

Nutrition Information

- ➢ Calories: 280
- ➢ Protein: 25g
- ➢ Carbohydrates: 20g
- ➢ Fat: 12g
- ➢ Fiber: 4g
- ➢ Cook Time: 20 minutes
- ➢ Prep Time: 15 minutes

Vegetable and Chicken Skewers

INGREDIENTS

- 1 lb boneless, skinless chicken breast (cut into cubes)
- 2 bell peppers (sliced)
- 1 red onion (sliced)
- Cherry tomatoes
- 3 tablespoons olive oil
- 1 teaspoon dried rosemary
- 1 teaspoon paprika
- Salt and pepper to taste

PREPARATION

- Preheat grill or oven broiler.
- In a bowl, combine chicken cubes, bell peppers, red onion, and cherry tomatoes.
- In a separate bowl, mix olive oil, dried rosemary, paprika, salt, and pepper.
- Thread the chicken and vegetables onto skewers and brush with the olive oil mixture.
- Grill or broil for 10-12 minutes, turning occasionally until chicken is cooked through and vegetables are tender.

Nutrition Information

- Calories: 320
- Protein: 28g
- Carbohydrates: 15g
- Fat: 16g
- Fiber: 4g
- Cook Time: 15 minutes
- Prep Time: 20 minutes

Eggplant and Chickpea Curry

INGREDIENTS

- 1 large eggplant (cubed)
- 1 can (15 oz) chickpeas (drained and rinsed)
- 1 onion (chopped)
- 3 tomatoes (chopped)
- 2 tablespoons curry powder
- 1 teaspoon turmeric
- 1 can (14 oz) coconut milk
- 2 tablespoons olive oil
- Salt and pepper to taste

PREPARATION

- In a large pot, sauté onions in olive oil until softened.
- Add eggplant and cook until browned.
- Stir in curry powder and turmeric, then add chopped tomatoes and chickpeas.
- Pour in coconut milk and let it simmer for 20-25 minutes.
- Season with salt and pepper before serving over brown rice or quinoa.

Nutrition Information

- Calories: 350
- Protein: 12g
- Carbohydrates: 40g
- Fat: 18g
- Fiber: 12g
- Cook Time: 30 minutes
- Prep Time: 15 minutes

Spinach and Feta Stuffed Chicken

INGREDIENTS

- ❖ 4 boneless, skinless chicken breasts
- ❖ 2 cups fresh spinach (chopped)
- ❖ 1/2 cup feta cheese (crumbled)
- ❖ 1 tablespoon olive oil
- ❖ 1 teaspoon dried oregano
- ❖ 2 cloves garlic (minced)
- ❖ Salt and pepper to taste

PREPARATION

- ❖ Preheat oven to 375°F (190°C).
- ❖ In a pan, sauté spinach and garlic in olive oil until wilted. Remove from heat and stir in feta.
- ❖ Cut a pocket into each chicken breast and stuff with the spinach and feta mixture.
- ❖ Sprinkle dried oregano, salt, and pepper over the chicken.
- ❖ Bake for 25-30 minutes or until the chicken is cooked through.

Nutrition Information

- ➢ Calories: 290
- ➢ Protein: 32g
- ➢ Carbohydrates: 2g
- ➢ Fat: 17g
- ➢ Fiber: 1g
- ➢ Cook Time: 30 minutes
- ➢ Prep Time: 20 minutes

Quinoa and Black Bean Stuffed Peppers

INGREDIENTS

- ❖ 4 bell peppers (halved and seeds removed)
- ❖ 1 cup quinoa (cooked)
- ❖ 1 can (15 oz) black beans (drained and rinsed)
- ❖ 1 cup corn kernels
- ❖ 1 cup salsa
- ❖ 1 teaspoon cumin
- ❖ 1/2 teaspoon chili powder
- ❖ 1/2 cup shredded cheddar cheese
- ❖ Fresh cilantro for garnish

PREPARATION

- ❖ Preheat oven to 375°F (190°C).
- ❖ In a bowl, mix cooked quinoa, black beans, corn, salsa, cumin, and chili powder.
- ❖ Stuff each pepper half with the quinoa mixture and place in a baking dish.
- ❖ Sprinkle shredded cheddar cheese over the peppers.
- ❖ Bake for 25-30 minutes or until the peppers are tender.
- ❖ Garnish with fresh cilantro before serving.

Nutrition Information

- ➢ Calories: 320
- ➢ Protein: 15g
- ➢ Carbohydrates: 50g
- ➢ Fat: 8g
- ➢ Fiber: 10g
- ➢ Cook Time: 30 minutes
- ➢ Prep Time: 20 minutes

Cucumber and Avocado Bites

INGREDIENTS

- 1 cucumber, sliced
- 1 ripe avocado, mashed
- Cherry tomatoes, halved
- Fresh basil leaves
- Olive oil
- Salt and pepper to taste

PREPARATION

- Lay out cucumber slices on a platter.
- Top each slice with a dollop of mashed avocado.
- Add a halved cherry tomato on each cucumber-avocado bite.
- Garnish with fresh basil leaves.
- Drizzle olive oil over the bites and season with salt and pepper.
- Serve chilled.

Nutrition Information

- Calories: 75
- Protein: 2g
- Fiber: 3g
- Healthy Fats: 6g
- Carbohydrates: 5g
- Cook Time: 10 minutes
- Prep Time: 15 minutes

Greek Yogurt Parfait with Berries

INGREDIENTS

- 1 cup Greek yogurt (unsweetened)
- Mixed berries (blueberries, strawberries, raspberries)
- Honey or stevia for sweetness
- Granola (optional)

PREPARATION

- In a glass or bowl, layer Greek yogurt.
- Add a generous handful of mixed berries.
- Drizzle honey or sprinkle stevia for sweetness.
- Optionally, top with granola for crunch.
- Repeat layers.
- Enjoy this delightful parfait.

Nutrition Information

- Calories: 180
- Protein: 15g
- Fiber: 5g
- Carbohydrates: 25g
- Healthy Fats: 3g
- Cook Time: 5 minutes
- Prep Time: 10 minutes

Baked Sweet Potato Chips

INGREDIENTS

- ❖ 2 sweet potatoes, thinly sliced
- ❖ Olive oil
- ❖ Paprika
- ❖ Garlic powder
- ❖ Sea salt

PREPARATION

- ❖ Preheat oven to 375°F (190°C).
- ❖ Toss sweet potato slices with olive oil, paprika, and garlic powder.
- ❖ Arrange on a baking sheet.
- ❖ Bake for 20-25 minutes until crisp.
- ❖ Sprinkle with sea salt.

Nutrition Information

- ➤ Calories: 120
- ➤ Protein: 2g
- ➤ Fiber: 4g
- ➤ Carbohydrates: 25g
- ➤ Healthy Fats: 2g
- ➤ Cook Time: 25 minutes
- ➤ Prep Time: 15 minutes

Caprese Skewers

INGREDIENTS

- ❖ Fresh mozzarella balls
- ❖ Cherry tomatoes
- ❖ Fresh basil leaves
- ❖ Balsamic glaze
- ❖ Olive oil
- ❖ Salt and pepper to taste

PREPARATION

- ❖ Thread mozzarella balls, cherry tomatoes, and basil leaves onto small skewers.
- ❖ Arrange the skewers on a serving platter.
- ❖ Drizzle with balsamic glaze and olive oil.
- ❖ Sprinkle with salt and pepper.
- ❖ Serve as a refreshing and flavorful snack.

Nutrition Information

- ➤ Calories: 90
- ➤ Protein: 6g
- ➤ Fiber: 1g
- ➤ Carbohydrates: 3g
- ➤ Healthy Fats: 6g
- ➤ Cook Time: 10 minutes
- ➤ Prep Time: 15 minutes

Almond and Berry Smoothie

INGREDIENTS

- ❖ 1 cup almond milk
- ❖ Handful of mixed berries (strawberries, blueberries, raspberries)
- ❖ 1 tablespoon almond butter
- ❖ Ice cubes
- ❖ Stevia or honey for sweetness

PREPARATION

- ❖ Blend almond milk, mixed berries, almond butter, and ice cubes until smooth.
- ❖ Add stevia or honey to taste.
- ❖ Pour into a glass and enjoy this nutrient-packed smoothie.

Nutrition Information

- ➢ Calories: 150
- ➢ Protein: 5g
- ➢ Fiber: 4g
- ➢ Carbohydrates: 20g
- ➢ Healthy Fats: 7g
- ➢ Cook Time: 5 minutes
- ➢ Prep Time: 8 minutes

Zucchini Hummus Roll-Ups

INGREDIENTS

- ❖ Zucchini strips
- ❖ Hummus
- ❖ Roasted red peppers, sliced
- ❖ Spinach leaves

PREPARATION

- ❖ Spread hummus over zucchini strips.
- ❖ Place roasted red pepper slices and spinach leaves on top.
- ❖ Roll up each strip.
- ❖ Secure with toothpicks and serve.

Nutrition Information

- ➢ Protein: 3g
- ➢ Fiber: 2g
- ➢ Carbohydrates: 10g
- ➢ Healthy Fats: 4g
- ➢ Cook Time: 8 minutes
- ➢ Prep Time: 12 minutes

Tuna and Avocado Lettuce Wraps

INGREDIENTS

- ❖ Canned tuna, drained
- ❖ Avocado, mashed
- ❖ Bibb lettuce leaves
- ❖ Cherry tomatoes, halved
- ❖ Lemon juice
- ❖ Salt and pepper to taste

PREPARATION

- ❖ In a bowl, mix tuna with mashed avocado.
- ❖ Season with lemon juice, salt, and pepper.
- ❖ Spoon the tuna-avocado mixture onto Bibb lettuce leaves.
- ❖ Top with halved cherry tomatoes.
- ❖ Wrap and secure with toothpicks for a satisfying, low-carb snack.

Nutrition Information

- ➢ Calories: 120
- ➢ Protein: 15g
- ➢ Fiber: 4g
- ➢ Carbohydrates: 6g
- ➢ Healthy Fats: 6g
- ➢ Cook Time: 10 minutes
- ➢ Prep Time: 15 minutes

Apple and Almond Butter Sandwiches

INGREDIENTS

- ❖ Apple slices
- ❖ Almond butter
- ❖ Chia seeds (optional)
- ❖ Cinnamon

PREPARATION

- ❖ Spread almond butter between two apple slices.
- ❖ Optionally, sprinkle chia seeds and cinnamon.
- ❖ Press the slices together to make a delicious sandwich.

Nutrition Information

- ➢ Calories: 100
- ➢ Protein: 2g
- ➢ Fiber: 4g
- ➢ Carbohydrates: 12g
- ➢ Healthy Fats: 5g
- ➢ Cook Time: 5 minutes
- ➢ Prep Time: 8 minutes

Quinoa Salad Cups

INGREDIENTS

- Cooked quinoa
- Diced cucumbers
- Cherry tomatoes, quartered
- Feta cheese, crumbled
- Olive oil and lemon dressing
- Fresh mint leaves

PREPARATION

- Mix quinoa, cucumbers, tomatoes, and feta in a bowl.
- Drizzle with olive oil and lemon dressing.
- Spoon the mixture into small lettuce cups.
- Garnish with fresh mint leaves.

Nutrition Information

- Calories: 150
- Protein: 5g
- Fiber: 3g
- Carbohydrates: 20g
- Healthy Fats: 6g
- Cook Time: 15 minutes
- Prep Time: 20 minutes

Dark Chocolate-Dipped Strawberries

INGREDIENTS

- Fresh strawberries
- Dark chocolate (70% cocoa or higher)
- Chopped nuts (optional)

PREPARATION

- Melt dark chocolate in a heatproof bowl.
- Dip each strawberry into the melted chocolate.
- Optionally, roll in chopped nuts.
- Place on parchment paper and let them cool.

Nutrition Information

- Calories: 60
- Protein: 1g
- Fiber: 2g
- Carbohydrates: 8g
- Healthy Fats: 3g
- Cook Time: 10 minutes
- Prep Time: 15 minutes

Dessert Recipes Suitable for a Diabetic and Renal Diet

Cinnamon-Spiced Baked Apples

INGREDIENTS

- ❖ 4 medium-sized apples, cored and halved
- ❖ 1 tablespoon ground cinnamon
- ❖ 1 tablespoon unsalted butter (or a suitable butter substitute)
- ❖ 2 tablespoons chopped walnuts (optional)
- ❖ 1 tablespoon sugar substitute

PREPARATION

- ❖ Preheat the oven to 350°F (175°C).
- ❖ In a bowl, mix cinnamon and sugar substitute.
- ❖ Place apples in a baking dish, sprinkle with the cinnamon mixture, and dot with butter.
- ❖ Bake for 25-30 minutes until apples are tender.
- ❖ Optional: Sprinkle chopped walnuts before serving.

Nutrition Information

- ➢ Calories: 120
- ➢ Carbohydrates: 25g
- ➢ Protein: 1g
- ➢ Fat: 3g
- ➢ Fiber: 5g
- ➢ Sodium: 2mg
- ➢ Cook Time: 25-30 minutes
- ➢ Prep Time: 10 minutes

Chia Seed Pudding with Berries

INGREDIENTS

- ❖ 1/4 cup chia seeds
- ❖ 1 cup unsweetened almond milk
- ❖ 1 teaspoon vanilla extract
- ❖ 1 tablespoon sugar substitute
- ❖ 1/2 cup mixed berries (blueberries, strawberries)

PREPARATION

- ❖ In a bowl, mix chia seeds, almond milk, vanilla extract, and sugar substitute.
- ❖ Refrigerate for at least 2 hours or overnight, stirring occasionally.
- ❖ Before serving, top with mixed berries.

Nutrition Information

- ➢ Calories: 120
- ➢ Carbohydrates: 15g
- ➢ Protein: 4g
- ➢ Fat: 5g
- ➢ Fiber: 8g
- ➢ Sodium: 10mg
- ➢ Cook Time: 2 hours (chilling time)
- ➢ Prep Time: 5 minutes

Avocado Chocolate Mousse

INGREDIENTS

- ❖ 2 ripe avocados
- ❖ 1/4 cup unsweetened cocoa powder
- ❖ 1/4 cup sugar substitute
- ❖ 1 teaspoon vanilla extract
- ❖ Pinch of salt

PREPARATION

- ❖ Blend avocados, cocoa powder, sugar substitute, vanilla extract, and salt until smooth.
- ❖ Chill in the refrigerator for 1-2 hours before serving.

Nutrition Information

- ➢ Calories: 150
- ➢ Carbohydrates: 12g
- ➢ Protein: 3g
- ➢ Fat: 12g
- ➢ Fiber: 7g
- ➢ Sodium: 5mg
- ➢ Cook Time: 1-2 hours (chilling time)
- ➢ Prep Time: 10 minutes

Strawberry Banana Frozen Yogurt Popsicles

INGREDIENTS

- ❖ 1 cup fresh strawberries, hulled
- ❖ 1 ripe banana
- ❖ 1 cup Greek yogurt (unsweetened)
- ❖ 2 tablespoons honey or sugar substitute

PREPARATION

- ❖ In a blender, combine strawberries, banana, Greek yogurt, and honey.
- ❖ Blend until smooth.
- ❖ Pour the mixture into popsicle molds and freeze for at least 4 hours.

Nutrition Information

- ➢ Calories: 80
- ➢ Carbohydrates: 16g
- ➢ Protein: 3g
- ➢ Fat: 1g
- ➢ Fiber: 2g
- ➢ Sodium: 20mg
- ➢ Cook Time: 4 hours (freezing time)
- ➢ Prep Time: 10 minutes

Vanilla Almond Flour Cookies

INGREDIENTS

- 1 cup almond flour
- 1/4 cup unsalted butter (or a suitable butter substitute), softened
- 1/4 cup sugar substitute
- 1 large egg
- 1 teaspoon vanilla extract

PREPARATION

- Preheat the oven to 350°F (175°C).
- In a bowl, cream together softened butter and sugar substitute.
- Add the egg and vanilla extract, mixing well.
- Gradually add almond flour, stirring until combined.
- Scoop onto a baking sheet and flatten with a fork.
- Bake for 10-12 minutes until edges are golden.

Nutrition Information

- Calories: 90
- Carbohydrates: 3g
- Protein: 2g
- Fat: 8g
- Fiber: 1g
- Sodium: 25mg
- Cook Time: 10-12 minutes
- Prep Time: 15 minutes

Peach and Blueberry Compote with Almond Crumble

INGREDIENTS

- 2 ripe peaches, peeled and sliced
- 1 cup blueberries
- 1 tablespoon lemon juice
- 2 tablespoons sugar substitute
- 1/4 cup almond flour
- 2 tablespoons chopped almonds
- 1 tablespoon unsalted butter (or a suitable butter substitute)

PREPARATION

- In a saucepan, combine peaches, blueberries, lemon juice, and sugar substitute.
- Simmer over low heat until fruits soften and release their juices.
- In a separate bowl, mix almond flour, chopped almonds, and softened butter to form a crumble.
- Serve the warm fruit compote topped with almond crumble.

Nutrition Information

- Calories: 110
- Carbohydrates: 15g
- Protein: 2g
- Fat: 6g
- Fiber: 3g
- Sodium: 5mg
- Cook Time: 15 minutes
- Prep Time: 10 minutes

Coconut-Lime Avocado Sorbet

INGREDIENTS

- ❖ 2 ripe avocados
- ❖ 1/2 cup coconut milk (unsweetened)
- ❖ Zest and juice of 2 limes
- ❖ 1/4 cup sugar substitute
- ❖ 1/4 teaspoon coconut extract (optional)

PREPARATION

- ❖ Blend avocados, coconut milk, lime zest, lime juice, sugar substitute, and coconut extract until smooth.
- ❖ Pour the mixture into a shallow dish and freeze for 3-4 hours, stirring every hour.

Nutrition Information

- ➢ Calories: 140
- ➢ Carbohydrates: 8g
- ➢ Protein: 2g
- ➢ Fat: 11g
- ➢ Fiber: 4g
- ➢ Sodium: 5mg
- ➢ Cook Time: 3-4 hours (freezing time)
- ➢ Prep Time: 15 minutes

Walnut and Date Energy Bites

INGREDIENTS

- ❖ 1 cup pitted dates
- ❖ 1 cup walnuts
- ❖ 1 tablespoon chia seeds
- ❖ 1/2 teaspoon cinnamon
- ❖ Pinch of salt

PREPARATION

- ❖ In a food processor, blend dates, walnuts, chia seeds, cinnamon, and salt until a sticky dough forms.
- ❖ Roll into bite-sized balls and refrigerate for at least 30 minutes before serving.

Nutrition Information

- ➢ Calories: 90
- ➢ Carbohydrates: 12g
- ➢ Protein: 2g
- ➢ Fat: 5g
- ➢ Fiber: 2g
- ➢ Sodium: 1mg
- ➢ Cook Time: 30 minutes (chilling time)
- ➢ Prep Time: 10 minutes

Raspberry Almond Chia Pudding Parfait

INGREDIENTS

- ❖ 1/4 cup chia seeds
- ❖ 1 cup unsweetened almond milk
- ❖ 1 teaspoon almond extract
- ❖ 1 tablespoon sugar substitute
- ❖ 1/2 cup fresh raspberries

PREPARATION

- ❖ Mix chia seeds, almond milk, almond extract, and sugar substitute. Refrigerate for at least 2 hours.
- ❖ In serving glasses, layer chia pudding with fresh raspberries

Nutrition Information

- ➢ Calories: 100
- ➢ Carbohydrates: 13g
- ➢ Protein: 3g
- ➢ Fat: 5g
- ➢ Fiber: 7g
- ➢ Sodium: 10mg
- ➢ Cook Time: 2 hours (chilling time)
- ➢ Prep Time: 5 minutes

Pistachio and Orange Dark Chocolate Bark

INGREDIENTS

- ❖ 1/2 cup shelled pistachios, chopped
- ❖ Zest of 1 orange
- ❖ 1/2 cup dark chocolate (70% cocoa or higher), melted
- ❖ 1 tablespoon sugar substitute

PREPARATION

- ❖ Mix chopped pistachios, orange zest, and sugar substitute.
- ❖ Spread melted dark chocolate onto a parchment-lined tray.
- ❖ Sprinkle the pistachio mixture on top and refrigerate until set.
- ❖ Break into pieces before serving.

Nutrition Information

- ➢ Calories: 120
- ➢ Carbohydrates: 10g
- ➢ Protein: 3g
- ➢ Fat: 8g
- ➢ Fiber: 2g
- ➢ Sodium: 5mg
- ➢ Cook Time: 1 hour (chilling time)
- ➢ Prep Time: 15 minutes

Chapter 5

MEAL PLANNING AND PORTION CONTROL

Creating Balanced Meals for Seniors

Our nutritional requirements change as we get older, making a balanced diet more and more important for general health. It is impossible to overestimate the importance of preparing wholesome, well-rounded meals for elders. We will examine the skill of preparing balanced meals that are specially targeted to the special requirements of seniors in this investigation of nutrition for the golden years.

Physiological changes brought about by aging need for a careful approach to diet. A diet high in vital nutrients is necessary due to factors such as a slower metabolism, reduced muscular mass, and probable health issues. Creating well-balanced meals is not only a matter of taste; it is a calculated decision that will help you stay healthy, avoid illness, and maintain your energy for years to come.

A varied range of nutrients is ensured by skillfully combining different food categories to create balanced meals. A senior's plate should be constructed with the following pillars at its base:

Fruits and Vegetables: Choose a rainbow of colors, since each shade represents a particular combination of vitamins and minerals. They provide vital fiber, antioxidants, and minerals needed to sustain optimum health.

Protein: Include foods high in lean protein, such as fish, chicken, beans, and tofu. Protein is essential for immune system support, tissue regeneration, and the maintenance of muscular mass.

Whole Grains: Choose whole wheat bread, brown rice, and quinoa among other whole grains. These include fiber, complex carbs, and a slow-release energy source—all of which are very helpful for seniors trying to keep their blood sugar levels stable.

Dairy or Dairy Substitutes: Incorporate calcium and vitamin D sources to support healthy bones. Dairy products with low or no fat and fortified plant-based substitutes may help reach the daily required consumption.

Healthy Fats: Include foods high in unsaturated fats, such as olive oil, avocados, nuts, and seeds. These fats promote general cardiovascular health, assist in nutrition absorption, and enhance cognitive function.

Mindful Eating and Portion Control:

Portion control is another important aspect of well-balanced meals. As we age, our metabolism slows down, so controlling our portions is essential to avoiding unintended weight gain. Healthy eating habits, such as enjoying each meal and paying attention to fullness signs, may promote a positive connection with food.

Hydration Is Important:

A well-rounded meal plan would be inadequate if it did not highlight how important it is to drink enough water. Dehydration may make typical problems experienced by seniors worse, such as constipation and impaired renal function. To maintain adequate hydration levels, promote the intake of water, herbal teas, and hydrating meals like fruits and vegetables.

Due to health issues like diabetes or renal problems, many seniors may have dietary limitations. In these situations, creating balanced meals requires paying close attention to salt content, and carbohydrate consumption, and following nutritional recommendations. Seeking advice from licensed dietitians or healthcare experts might provide tailored recommendations to meet specific requirements.
Meal preparation may make a big difference for elders. It makes meal preparation easier and guarantees a steady consumption of nutrient-dense meals. When fresh produce is more difficult to come by, think about cooking in larger quantities, using pre-cut veggies, and choosing frozen fruits and vegetables instead. This strategy encourages nutrition and convenience.

Balanced meals include the social and emotional aspects of eating as well as the nutritional component. Seniors may create a feeling of community and pleasure at the dinner table by being encouraged to eat with friends and family. This social interaction improves general well-being and elevates the eating experience above and beyond the nutritional value of the meal.

Making healthy meals for older citizens is a multifaceted process that incorporates culinary creativity, mindfulness, and nutritional science. It's an investment in life, good health, and the happiness that comes from enjoying each mouthful of a delicious, nutritious meal. Seniors may have meaningful, healthy, and energetic lives as long as we embrace the art of balanced nutrition.

Importance of Portion Control in Managing Diabetes and Kidney Disease

One crucial but sometimes disregarded element in the complex dance of controlling diabetes and renal disease is portion management. Since portion control is a keystone that leads people through the maze of health management, it is critical to comprehend the tremendous effect it has on the delicate balance needed for those who are coping with these two common disorders.

Before exploring the importance of portion management, let us examine the complex relationship between diabetes and renal disease. Over time, diabetes, a disorder characterized by decreased insulin activity, may cause significant damage to the kidneys. Increased blood sugar levels may put more strain on the kidneys, which remove waste and extra fluid from the blood.

The interplay among these disorders emphasizes how important it is to have a holistic approach to health care. One of the main components of this method is portion management, which is essential for controlling blood sugar and protecting renal function.

Finding the right balance between restriction and nutrition is one of the main issues facing people with diabetes and renal disease. Portion management serves as a safety measure, limiting the amount of food consumed in excess that might worsen blood sugar increases or put undue pressure on the kidneys.

Imagine this situation: if portion sizes are not closely supervised, a well-meaning dinner that includes wholesome ingredients may unintentionally turn into a health risk. People may enjoy a wide range of meals without sacrificing their health by controlling their portion sizes, which creates a harmonic balance between gastronomic pleasure and dietary responsibility.

It is impossible to emphasize how crucial portion control is to blood sugar management for those with diabetes. Large servings may cause a sudden surge of glucose into the blood, making it more difficult for the body to properly control blood sugar levels. People may improve their glycemic control by reducing their chance of experiencing abrupt rises in blood sugar by controlling their portion sizes.

Portion management becomes an effective strategy for kidney preservation when it comes to diseases like kidney disease when the kidneys are already under stress. Large meals have the potential to accelerate the course of renal disease by raising blood pressure and adding to the load on the kidneys. Adopting portion control may help people reduce the amount of strain on their kidneys, which can help them perform at their best and perhaps slow down the progression of renal problems.

Effective Portion Control Techniques: Recognizing the significance of portion control is one thing, but putting it into practice daily is quite another. The following are doable methods for smoothly incorporating portion restriction into daily life:

Plate Method: To offer a visual indication for balanced quantities, divide the plate into areas for veggies, lean proteins, and carbs.

Measuring Tools: Accurately calculating portions with the use of food scales and measuring cups enables people to make well-informed decisions.

Mindful Eating: By being aware of your body's signals of hunger and fullness, you may eat mindfully and avoid overindulging.

More Regular, Smaller Meals: Choosing more regular, smaller meals throughout the day will help control blood sugar levels and lessen the strain on the kidneys.

Nutritional Guidance: Consulting with dietitians or medical specialists may provide tailored advice on portion sizes that take into account each person's unique health requirements.

The Way Ahead: Portion management shows up as a compass in the complex web of controlling diabetes and kidney disease, pointing people in the direction of a more balanced and healthful lifestyle. Instead of focusing on deprivation, people should be empowered to enjoy life to the fullest while protecting their health.

Let's embrace portion management as a liberating force that allows us to take control of our health rather than as a limitation as we go forward. We can untangle the complexity of kidney disease and diabetes by making thoughtful and educated decisions, opening the door to a happy and rewarding future.

Chapter 6

LIFESTYLE TIPS FOR SENIORS WITH DIABETES AND KIDNEY DISEASE

Exercise and Physical Activity Recommendations

It takes a careful and comprehensive strategy to manage diabetes and renal disease together throughout your senior years. Including regular exercise and physical activity in your daily routine is a crucial component of this trip. The transforming power of movement becomes more and more apparent when we go into the topic of lifestyle suggestions for seniors who are dealing with chronic health concerns.

Exercise is a powerful tool for improving general well-being, especially for seniors with diabetes and renal illness. Regular physical exercise supports the maintenance of good kidney function in addition to helping regulate blood sugar levels. The advantages touch on aspects of mental and emotional well-being in addition to physical health.

Starting a fitness regimen may seem intimidating to seniors, but the secret is to discover sustainable and fun activities. Easy workouts like swimming, strolling, or low-impact aerobics may be great places to start. Engaging in these exercises not only improves cardiovascular health but also builds muscle mass, which helps control diabetes.

Importantly, exercise is an effective way to control weight, which is essential for managing diabetes and renal disease. Even a small amount of weight loss may have a big impact on insulin sensitivity and lessen renal strain. To customize an exercise program that fits each person's unique demands and limits, it is essential to speak with healthcare specialists.

Beyond the obvious health advantages, regular exercise is essential for lowering stress, worry, and depression—all of which are frequent companions on the path to chronic disease. Playing games that make you happy and give you a feeling of success helps you maintain a positive outlook, which is essential for dealing with the difficulties that come with kidney and diabetes.

Essentially, including physical activity in the lives of elderly individuals suffering from diabetes and renal disease is essential for a better and more energetic future. It's an homage to the body's tenacity and a celebration of the spirit that perseveres in the face of health difficulties. Put on your shoes, enjoy the feeling of movement, and allow the transforming potential of physical activity to light your journey toward overall well-being.

Stress Management Techniques

The day-to-day uncertainties that accompany health issues, dietary limitations, and drug management are sometimes a crossroads for seniors. Stress may become a silent enemy during this delicate balancing effort and exacerbate the effects of renal disease and diabetes. Given this, it becomes imperative to include stress management in day-to-day activities.

Above all, it has been shown that regular exercise is an effective way to combat stress. Endorphins are the body's natural stress relievers, and they may be released with easy activities tailored to individual capacities. Walking, light yoga, or tai chi are examples of exercises that improve physical health as well as mental peacefulness.

Another method for reducing stress is to engage in mindfulness techniques. Seniors may manage times of increased stress by using strategies including guided visualization, meditation, and deep breathing exercises. Seniors who engage in these techniques not only develop emotional resilience but also mental calmness, which enables them to face obstacles head-on.

Emotional well-being is greatly influenced by social relationships. Seniors may benefit from having a strong support system in place to help them cope with the emotional strain of managing chronic health concerns. This network can be established via family, friends, or community organizations. Connecting with others who have been there before and who can relate to your experiences, pleasures, and even worries may make you feel less alone and more like you belong.

This examination of lifestyle recommendations emphasizes how controlling diabetes and renal disease in older adults is intertwined. We not only treat the emotional elements of health but also help to create a senior community that is more resilient and empowered by incorporating stress management practices into everyday life. By engaging in these activities, we want to cultivate a robust and full life despite any obstacles that may come along, rather than having a stress-free existence.

Hydration and Its Role in Kidney Health

It is impossible to overestimate the significance of hydration for kidney function, as it is a basic component of good health in general. As a well-being advocate, I have personally seen the game-changing effects that adequate hydration can have on the delicate equilibrium of our body's internal systems, particularly the kidneys. The kidneys are essential for controlling blood pressure, filtering waste materials, and preserving fluid and electrolyte balance. Maintaining these processes and delaying the development of kidney-related problems need enough hydration.

Think of the kidneys as careful stewards, constantly filtering the blood to get rid of waste products and pollutants. Their steadfast quest to preserve homeostasis has water as its friend. Drinking enough water keeps the kidneys' blood supply strong, which enables the kidneys to perform their filtering function effectively. It's like giving the kidneys a constant flow of support so they can work at their best.

Staying hydrated is especially important for those who are managing both renal disease and diabetes. Diabetes may increase the risk of renal issues; therefore, monitoring fluid intake closely is essential. Dehydration may cause concentrated urine, which raises the risk of urinary tract infections and kidney stones—two undesirable allies on the road to recovery.

How much water, however, is enough? Individual needs—which are impacted by variables including age, weight, climate, and general health—are the source of the solution. Aiming for eight 8-ounce glasses of water or more each day is an excellent place to start as a general rule of thumb. It is always essential to get individualized suggestions from healthcare specialists based on unique health situations.

Staying hydrated is a simple yet effective strategy for maintaining kidney health. We consciously decide to nurture our bodies from the inside out every day. Thus, let the stream of clean, cool water serve as a reminder of the assistance we provide to our hardworking kidneys, preserving not only their operation but also our general health.

Chapter 7

MONITORING AND MANAGING BLOOD SUGAR LEVELS

Few pieces in the complex puzzle of diabetes management are as important as routinely checking blood sugar levels. Regular monitoring is more than just a habit for people with diabetes; it's a compass that directs their path to the best possible health and well-being. We'll delve into the nuances of blood sugar monitoring in this investigation, comprehending its critical role in managing diabetes and enabling people to take control of their health.

Importance of Regular Monitoring

Diabetes, a disorder that causes the body to be unable to properly manage blood sugar, necessitates close monitoring of one's blood sugar levels. Our cells need glucose, often known as blood sugar, as their main source of energy. However, diabetes throws off the bloodstream's delicate glucose balance, which might result in difficulties. Thus, routine monitoring becomes the primary component of diabetes care that is proactive.

Consider blood sugar monitoring as a window into the internal operations of your body. Every reading reveals crucial details about how your body uses glucose, providing an understanding of the efficiency of medication, exercise, and food choices. People may use this window to see patterns, trends, and possible triggers, which enables them to make well-informed changes to their diabetes treatment strategy.

Timely Interventions and Preventive Measures: Regular blood sugar monitoring is a proactive approach to preventing possible consequences, not only an observational one. Prompt actions predicated on blood sugar measurements enable people to make knowledgeable choices, averting the rise in glucose levels that may result in health complications. Being able to respond quickly is a valuable skill in managing diabetes, whether it is via food changes, medication adjustments, or lifestyle alterations.

Personalized Diabetes Management: Diabetes is a highly personalized illness since each person's body reacts differently to different stimuli. Frequent monitoring makes it possible to create diabetes care programs that are specifically suited to the requirements of each patient. A tailored approach is made possible by knowing how the body responds to certain meals, activities, or stresses. This empowers people with diabetes to feel in charge of their health.

Blood sugar monitoring helps people and their healthcare providers build a cooperative connection. Healthcare professionals may make individualized suggestions, modify medication doses, and provide focused counsel when blood sugar data is shared regularly. This collaboration is essential to reaching and maintaining ideal blood sugar management, which eventually improves long-term health outcomes.

Overcoming dread and Developing Confidence: For some people, the idea of routinely checking their blood sugar could be frightening. This dread and anxiety are sometimes accompanied by uncertainty or concern about possible swings. But it's crucial to see monitoring as an empowering tool rather than a cause for fear. Through regular monitoring, people may gain an awareness of their bodies, overcome fear, and feel in control of their diabetes care.

Technological Developments in Blood Sugar Monitoring: As a result of technological developments, the field of blood sugar monitoring has undergone substantial change. With real-time data and increased convenience, continuous glucose monitoring (CGM) systems, intelligent insulin pumps, and user-friendly glucometers have completely changed the monitoring procedure. By using these technologies, monitoring may be streamlined, made more accessible, and incorporated into day-to-day activities.

It is impossible to overestimate the significance of routine blood sugar monitoring in the treatment of diabetes. It acts as a compass, helping people navigate the ever-changing terrain of their health. People may take control of their health, tailor their diabetes treatment, and build a cooperative relationship with medical experts by seeing monitoring as a proactive step. Maintaining a regular blood sugar level is more than just a routine—it's a path toward resilience against diabetes, self-empowerment, and self-discovery. Therefore, let's embrace this trip with the information, tools, and willpower to confidently and gracefully traverse the cycles of health.

A complete strategy is necessary to navigate the complex terrain of diabetes and kidney disease, and medication management and adherence are essential components of this trip. As we examine this crucial aspect of health, it becomes clear that managing medications correctly is more than simply taking pills; it's a symphony of time, accuracy, and dedication that may profoundly affect a person's course in life.

For those who are juggling both diabetes and renal illness, prescription drugs are often the mainstay of their care. It becomes crucial to maintain a careful balance between insulin, oral hypoglycemics, and drugs that promote renal function. This dance calls for a customized road map created by medical experts who are aware of the subtleties of each person's unique health situation, not simply a prescription.

The key to managing these illnesses effectively is maintaining drug regimen adherence. Being consistent is a need rather than just a virtue. Missing doses or consuming food inconsistently may cause blood sugar levels to fluctuate, endangering kidney function as well as general health. The consequences of noncompliance are not limited to the here and now; they also have long-term effects that may hasten the advancement of these persistent illnesses.

Recognizing the connection between kidney function and diabetes is necessary to appreciate the significance of medication adherence. Critical to reducing the risks associated with these disorders are medications that maintain renal function, control blood pressure, and regulate blood glucose levels. To create a relationship where people take an active role in managing their own health, education and open communication with healthcare practitioners are vital.

Adherence goes beyond the pillbox, too. Supplementary medication management is achieved by lifestyle alterations, including food adjustments and consistent physical exercise. By embracing a feeling of agency in one's health journey, this holistic approach enables people to go beyond the position of passive receivers of prescriptions.

Medication management and adherence are interwoven with the treatment of diabetes and renal disease. People may forge a road toward a healthier, more vibrant future by understanding the need for consistency, communication, and cooperation with healthcare providers. With persistence and fortitude, people can negotiate this complex terrain

Diabetes and Kidney Disease Management

Kidney illness and diabetes often dance together in a way that has to be carefully managed to preserve optimum health. For those dealing with the twin difficulties of these diseases, it is essential to comprehend the nuances of this interaction.

Over time, diabetes, a chronic illness marked by high blood sugar, may cause serious harm to the kidneys. The kidneys are essential for eliminating waste from the blood, but they may get overworked as a result of diabetes's elevated blood sugar levels. renal damage from this ongoing strain may eventually result in renal disease.

An integrated strategy is necessary for the management of diabetes and renal disease. Tight control of blood sugar levels is the cornerstone of this approach. People who regularly check their blood glucose levels are better able to make educated decisions regarding their food, medications, and lifestyle choices. This is generally achieved by routine blood glucose testing.

Using a diet that is renal-friendly and meets the requirements of both illnesses is essential to this therapy. This usually entails cutting down on salt, limiting protein intake, and managing potassium and phosphorus levels. Adopting a low-carb diet is often advised as an efficient way to control diabetes and lessen the strain on the kidneys.

Maintaining enough hydration is essential for managing renal illness. An adequately hydrated body promotes kidney function, which aids in the effective removal of waste and pollutants. However, severe renal disease patients may need to reduce their fluid consumption, so it's important to find a careful balance.

Exercise regularly has a major positive impact on general well-being, independent of nutrition. Engaging in physical exercise is beneficial for controlling blood sugar levels and cardiovascular health, which is important for those who are managing diabetes and renal illness.

Most importantly, working together with medical specialists is essential. Effective management is based on regular check-ups, medication adherence, and open contact with healthcare practitioners. Knowing how diabetes and renal illness work

hand in hand gives people the ability to make wise decisions and encourages them
to take the initiative to lead healthier, more balanced lives.

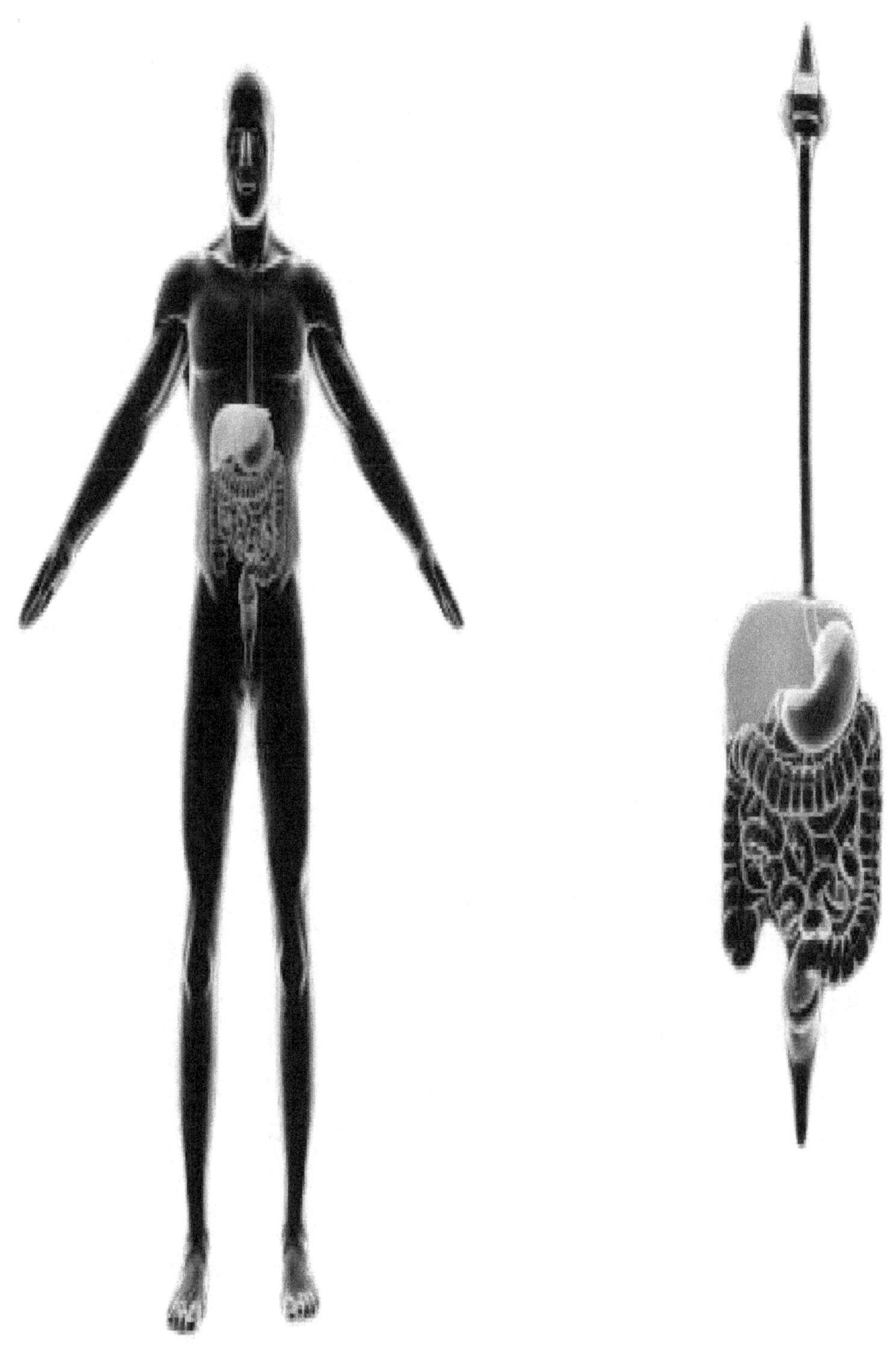

Conclusion

Diabetes Renal Diet Cookbook for Seniors: The Complete Seniors' Low Carb Guide to Managing Kidney Disease and Diabetes with 100+ Nourishing Recipes," comes to an end with this extensive manual. A deep feeling of hope and success fills me. Our journey together has included more than just gathering recipes and nutritional recommendations; it has also involved learning about empowerment, resilience, and the many possibilities for enhancing one's health.

We have explored the complex dance of controlling diabetes and renal illness in our beloved elders over these pages. We now know the subtleties of striking a balance between tastes, textures, and health needs as we have deciphered the secrets of low-carb, renal-friendly eating. The tales interwoven throughout each chapter are more than simply anecdotes; they are symbols of the unwavering perseverance of people who, equipped with information and resolve, take on health difficulties head-on.

This book is a travel companion, more than just a manual for achieving ideal well-being. I hope this resource has been helpful and encouraging to you, whether you are a senior wanting to improve your health, a caregiver hoping to assist a loved one, or a health enthusiast searching for mindful meals.

Recall that maintaining your health is a journey, not a destination, as we part ways. Everyday decisions we make about our diet, way of life, and mentality add to the fabric of our overall well-being. Accept the ability to alter things for the better and rejoice in your accomplishments, no matter how tiny.

Let this book serve, as evidence that living with diabetes and renal illness may be a tasty, fulfilling, and happy experience. I hope that the recipes on these pages will cheer your heart as well as fuel your body. Cheers to your perseverance, health, and a bright future full of energy and well-being. To the voyage ahead, cheers!

30 DAYS

MEAL PLAN

DAY 1	
BREAKFAST:	Greek Yogurt Parfait
LUNCH:	Grilled Chicken Salad
SNACK:	Fresh Fruit
DINNER:	Baked Salmon, Quinoa, Broccoli

DAY 2	
BREAKFAST:	Oatmeal with Berries
LUNCH:	Quinoa and Black Bean Bowl
SNACK:	Mixed Nuts
DINNER:	Vegetable Stir-Fry, Brown Rice

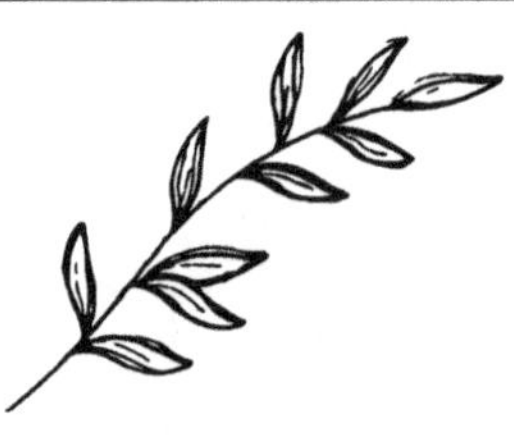
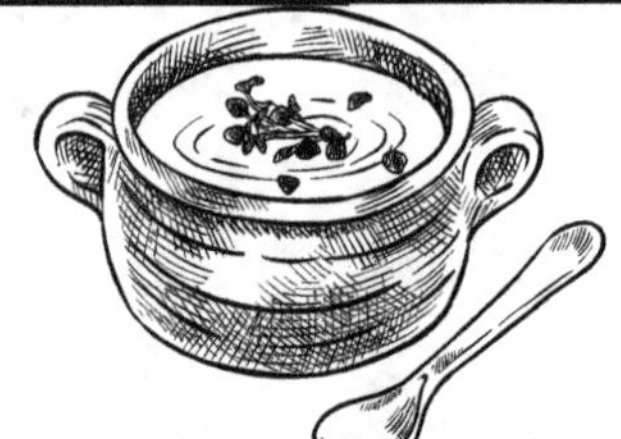
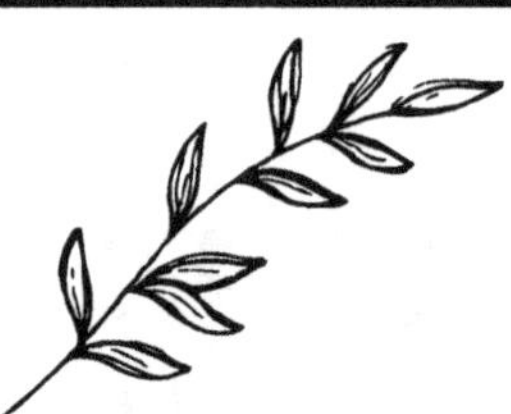

DAY 3	
BREAKFAST:	Scrambled Eggs, Avocado
LUNCH:	Chickpea Salad Wrap
SNACK:	Hummus with Veggies
DINNER:	Turkey Meatballs, Sweet Potato

DAY 4	
BREAKFAST:	Smoothie with Spinach
LUNCH:	Lentil Soup and Whole Grain Bread
SNACK:	Greek Yogurt with Berries
DINNER:	Grilled Shrimp, Couscous

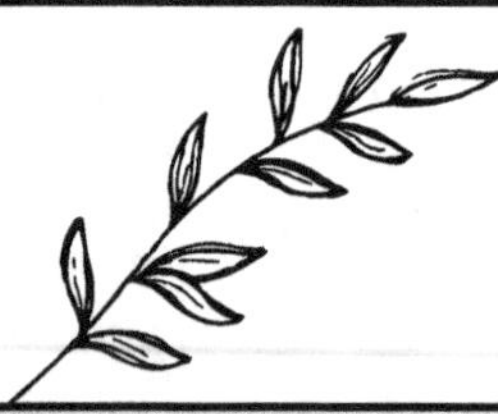
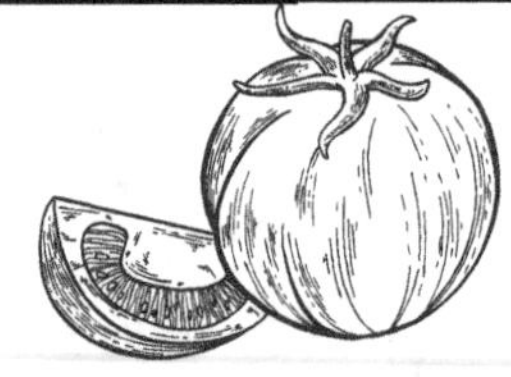
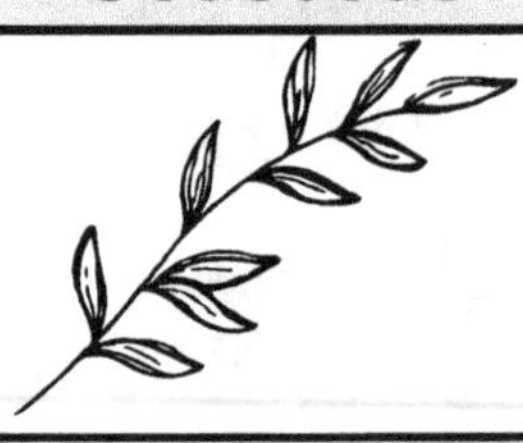

DAY 5	
BREAKFAST:	Whole Grain Toast, Peanut Butter
LUNCH:	Turkey and Veggie Wrap
SNACK:	Fresh Apple Slices
DINNER:	Chicken and Vegetable Skewers

DAY 6	
BREAKFAST:	Overnight Chia Pudding
LUNCH:	Quinoa Salad with Vinaigrette
SNACK:	Almond Butter with Celery
DINNER:	Baked Cod, Asparagus

DAY 7		DAY 8	
BREAKFAST:	Banana Walnut Muffins	**BREAKFAST:**	Spinach and Feta Omelette
LUNCH:	**Sweet Potato and Black Bean Bowl**	**LUNCH:**	Chicken Caesar Salad
SNACK:	Greek Yogurt with Granola	**SNACK:**	Cottage Cheese with Pineapple
DINNER:	Vegetarian Stir-Fried Tofu	**DINNER:**	Grilled Chicken, Quinoa, Broccoli

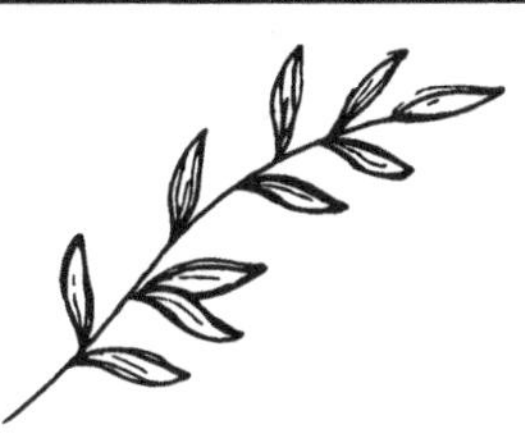
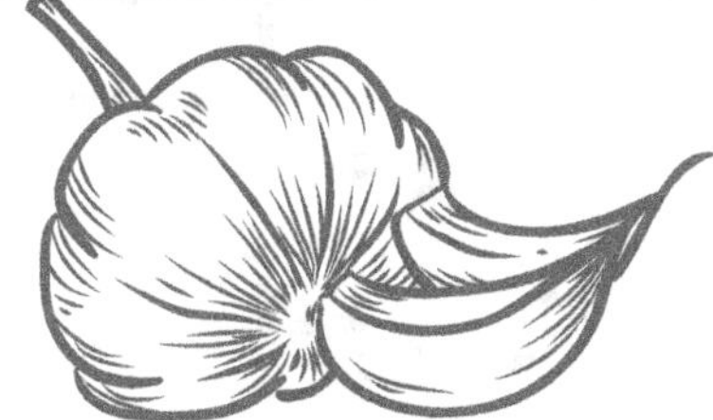
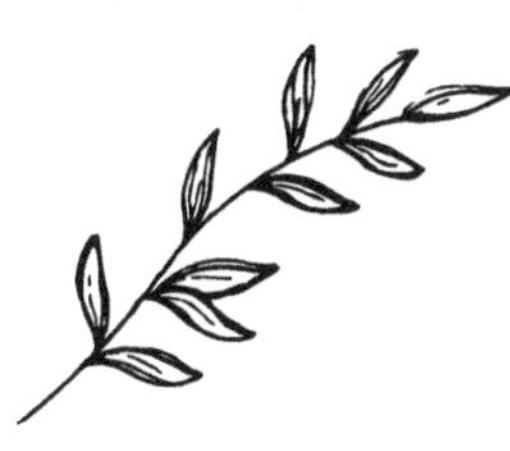

DAY 9		DAY 10	
BREAKFAST:	Acai Bowl with Granola	**BREAKFAST:**	Whole Grain Pancakes
LUNCH:	Veggie Wrap with Hummus	**LUNCH:**	Lentil Curry with Basmati Rice
SNACK:	Mixed Berries with Yogurt	**SNACK:**	Raw Veggies with Hummus
DINNER:	Baked Tilapia, Brown Rice	**DINNER:**	Beef Stir-Fry, Quinoa

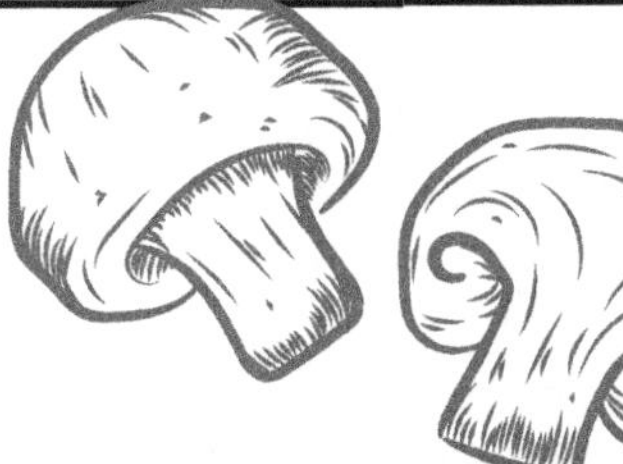

DAY 11		DAY 12	
BREAKFAST:	Avocado Toast with Egg	**BREAKFAST:**	Smoothie with Berries
LUNCH:	Mediterranean Quinoa Bowl	**LUNCH:**	Caprese Salad
SNACK:	Apple Slices with Almond Butter	**SNACK:**	Greek Yogurt with Walnuts
DINNER:	Turkey Chili with Cornbread	**DINNER:**	Grilled Salmon, Sweet Potato

DAY 13	
BREAKFAST: Chia Seed Smoothie Bowl	
LUNCH: Chickpea and Veggie Stir-Fry	
SNACK: Fresh Fruit Salad	
DINNER: Baked Chicken, Couscous	

DAY 14	
BREAKFAST: Breakfast Burrito	
LUNCH: Turkey and Avocado Wrap	
SNACK: Trail Mix	
DINNER: Quinoa Stuffed Bell Peppers	

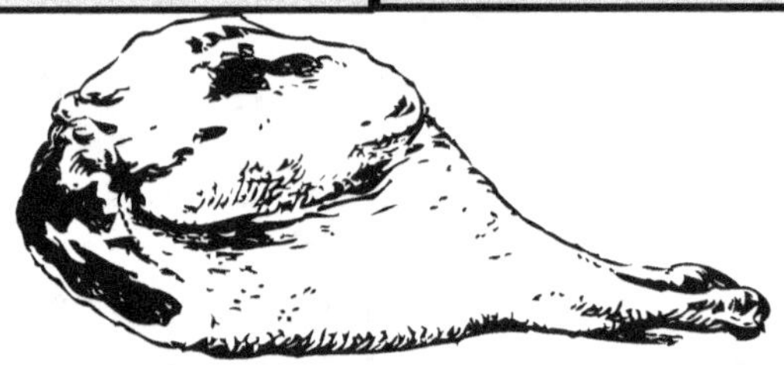

DAY 15	
BREAKFAST: Yogurt Parfait with Granola	
LUNCH: Quinoa Salad with Chickpeas	
SNACK: Cottage Cheese with Berries	
DINNER: Baked Cod, Brown Rice	

DAY 16	
BREAKFAST: Vegetable Omelette	
LUNCH: Lentil Soup and Whole Grain Bread	
SNACK: Greek Yogurt with Mango	
DINNER: Grilled Shrimp, Quinoa	

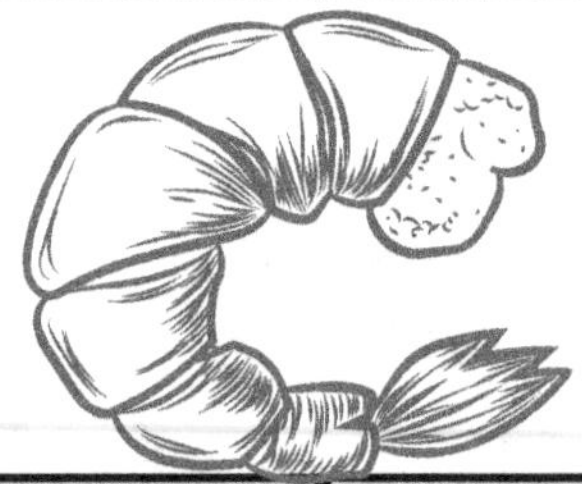

DAY 17	
BREAKFAST: Peanut Butter Banana Toast	
LUNCH: Turkey and Veggie Stir-Fry	
SNACK: Fresh Apple Slices	
DINNER: Chicken Fajitas, Black Beans	

DAY 18	
BREAKFAST: Blueberry Protein Pancakes	
LUNCH: Caprese Quinoa Bowl	
SNACK: Almond Butter with Carrots	
DINNER: Baked Tilapia, Sweet Potato	

DAY 19	
BREAKFAST: Smoothie Bowl with Kiwi	
LUNCH: Spinach and Feta Chickpea Salad	
SNACK: Mixed Nuts	
DINNER: Veggie Stir-Fried Tofu, Brown Rice	

DAY 20	
BREAKFAST: Breakfast Burrito Bowl	
LUNCH: Grilled Chicken Caesar Wrap	
SNACK: Hummus with Cucumber	
DINNER: Turkey Bolognese, Whole Wheat Pasta	

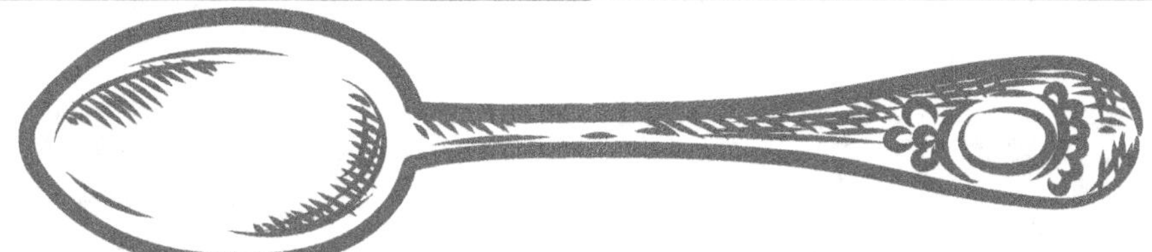

DAY 21	
BREAKFAST: Overnight Oats with Berries	
LUNCH: Quinoa and Black Bean Bowl	
SNACK: Greek Yogurt with Granola	
DINNER: Grilled Chicken, Quinoa, Broccoli	

DAY 22	
BREAKFAST: Acai Smoothie Bowl	
LUNCH: Chickpea Salad Wrap	
SNACK: Fresh Fruit Salad	
DINNER: Baked Cod, Asparagus	

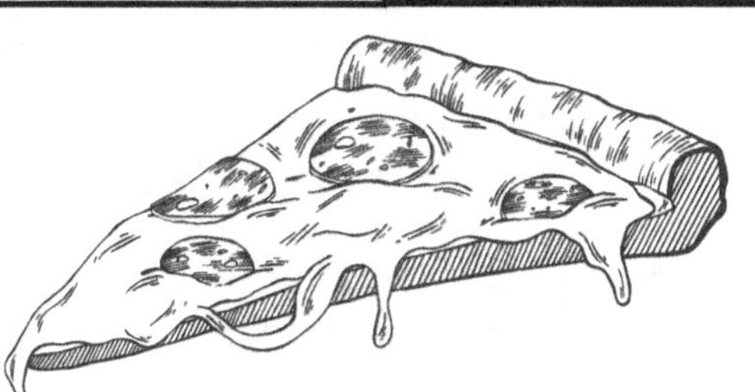

DAY 23	
BREAKFAST: Veggie Omelette	
LUNCH: Mediterranean Quinoa Bowl	
SNACK: Greek Yogurt with Walnuts	
DINNER: Grilled Shrimp, Sweet Potato	

DAY 24	
BREAKFAST: Chia Seed Pudding	
LUNCH: Lentil Curry with Basmati Rice	
SNACK: **Mixed Berries with Yogurt**	
DINNER: Turkey Chili with Cornbread	

DAY 25	DAY 26
BREAKFAST: Banana Walnut Muffins	**BREAKFAST:** Oatmeal with Almond Butter
LUNCH: Caprese Salad	**LUNCH:** Veggie Stir-Fried Tofu
SNACK: Cottage Cheese with Pineapple	**SNACK:** Hummus with Veggies
DINNER: Quinoa Stuffed Bell Peppers	**DINNER:** Chicken and Vegetable Skewers

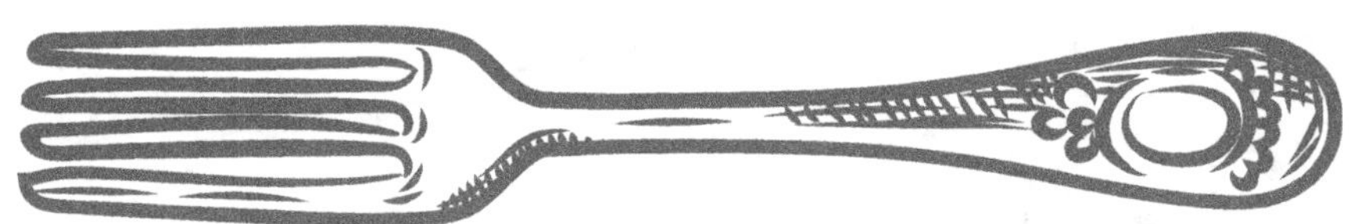

DAY 27	DAY 28
BREAKFAST: Smoothie with Spinach	**BREAKFAST:** Whole Grain Pancakes
LUNCH: Turkey and Avocado Wrap	**LUNCH:** Quinoa Salad with Vinaigrette
SNACK: Almond Butter with Celery	**SNACK:** Trail Mix
DINNER: Baked Salmon, Quinoa, Broccoli	**DINNER:** Beef Stir-Fry, Brown Rice

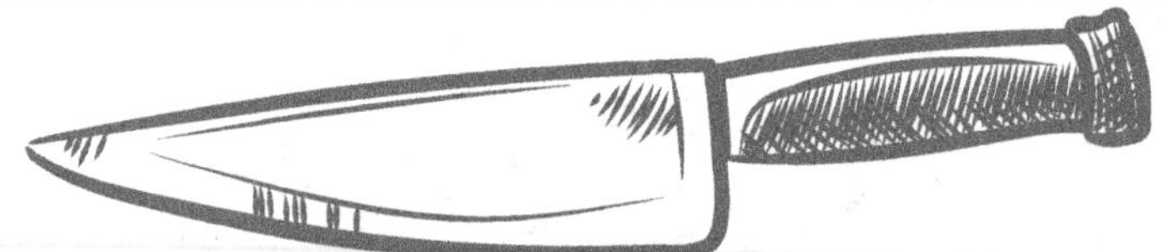

DAY 29	DAY 30
BREAKFAST: Avocado Toast with Egg	**BREAKFAST:** Greek Yogurt Parfait
LUNCH: Chickpea and Veggie Stir-Fry	**LUNCH:** Quinoa and Black Bean Bowl
SNACK: Greek Yogurt with Mango	**SNACK:** Fresh Apple Slices
DINNER: Grilled Chicken, Couscous	**DINNER:** Baked Tilapia, Brown Rice